To Betty, my wife

Oh, it's a long, long while from May to December
But the days grow short when you reach September . . .

. . . Oh, the days dwindle down to a precious few
September, November
And these few precious days I'll spend with you
These precious days I'll spend with you

— from *September Song*

Acknowledgments

I want to express my deep appreciation to my acquired unofficial "granddaughter" for the help she has given me with the computer in this endeavor. I am not computer literate. Eleanor Pomerat fixed all of my innumerable blunders which repeatedly occurred while I typed this manuscript. All it took was for me to yell, "Eleanor, I've goofed up again." She would come tripping up the stairs (God, how good it would be to trip up stairs again) and, without a single caustic remark, magically would make the monster start to work one more time.

This book would have never reached fruition without the help of my oldest daughter, Valerie. She would keep me going when I would be terribly tired of the whole affair. It was, "Dad, it is something that needs to be put out there." I can't remember when I last won an argument with her. Now that it is finished, I am truly glad she pushed me.

Then, I want to seriously thank my editor, Mia Tyler. She had the nerve to tell me that she couldn't read my handwriting. I was shocked, *shocked* that she said that. I vividly remember getting two As in penmanship in the second grade. Of course, that was seventy-six years ago. She was very tactful in correcting my southern English, and making me write in a way I don't remember learning in that same second grade. She made it up to me by drawing happy faces at the ends of my attempts at humor. When I became sentimental in a way she approved she would draw me hearts. She even drew me a heart when I said something was "scarce as hen's teeth."

Hippocratic Oath

I swear by Apollo Physician and Asclepius and Hygieia and Panaceia and all the gods and goddesses, making them my witnesses, that I will fulfill according to my ability and judgment.

To hold him who has taught me this art as equal to my parents and to live my life in partnership with him, and if he is in need of money to give him a share of mine, and to regard his offspring as equal to my brothers in male lineage and to teach them this art—if they desire to learn it—without fee and covenant; to give a share of precepts and oral instruction and all the other learning to my sons and to the sons of him who has instructed me and to pupils who have signed the covenant and have taken an oath according to the medical law, but no one else.

I will apply dietetic measures for the benefit of the sick according to my ability and judgment; I will keep them from harm and injustice.

I will neither give a deadly drug to anybody if asked for it, nor will I make a suggestion to this effect. Similarly I will not give to a woman an abortive remedy. In purity and holiness I will guard my life and my art.

I will not use the knife, not even on sufferers from stone, but will withdraw in favor of such men as are engaged in this work.

Whatever houses I may visit, I will come for the benefit of the sick, remaining free of all intentional injustice, of all mischief and in particular of sexual relations with both female and male persons, be they free or slaves.

What I may see or hear in the course of treatment or even outside of the treatment in regard to the life of men, which on no account one must spread abroad, I will keep to myself, holding such things shameful to be spoken about.

If I fulfill this oath and do not violate it, may it be granted to me to enjoy life and art, being honored with fame among all men for all time to come; if I transgress it and swear falsely, may the opposite of all this be my lot.

Table of Contents

Prologue

This is not in any way meant to be a detailed biography of my life. Every mortal is imperfect and does questionable things, and there is no need to chronicle them. Just say that in my more than over eighty years, and my penchant of always trying to make things better, I have made more than my share of dumb mistakes. There is absolutely no reason to dwell on them. I originally wrote these facts and experiences for my grandchildren and great-grandchildren in the form of a book describing my life and experiences. It was solely for their consumption and edification.

A great deal of this manuscript is taken unchanged from that first work, with only some family history deleted; it being of little interest to anyone except close friends and family members. I have written about some of my childhood memories, my educational experiences, and, particularly, my becoming a physician and the extremely interesting life that I lived because of that profession. I lived and practiced medicine in some of the best times of the medical profession, but then, perhaps I have lived a little too long. I have watched various inner and outside factors change my beloved profession so that now, in my opinion, there is a decline in the quality of day-to-day practice of medicine. A great deal of the humanity has vanished in the taking care of people with perceived illnesses, real or imagined. This humanity is the heart and soul of the "art of medicine" as described by Hippocrates. It is what makes the practice of medicine a profession and not a trade. We will discuss these matters later.

These pages document my decision to become a physician, the

various roads I traveled getting to be a physician, and the changes that have occurred in medicine along the way. These changes, in my opinion, include the lack of medical schools teaching their medical students throughout the four years of study that the care of the patient supersedes all other competing factors. The lack of emphasizing this teaching tenet is now becoming evident. A lack of patient responsibility for continuing care until a cure or failure of therapy is evident. It is becoming more frequently exhibited by some physicians. We will also delve into this later.

I thought about doing a lot of things in my early life. When the gas company was laying gas mains down the road in front of our house, I was determined that I was going to be a ditchdigger when I grew up. Later, I was going be a heavyweight boxing champion, an aviator, and a football coach. Eventually, I decided that I wanted to be a physician in a small town.

I have never varied from that desire since then, but many things, including a lot of my own making, have continually altered my achieving that personal goal in my life. As you will see, I have always demonstrated an inability to say "no" to friends and acquaintances. This has often led me away from my intended life. However, it did allow me to be in places and in circumstances where I was associated with first-time events in medicine and in the world. As a result, I became acquainted with some remarkable individuals and became a part of medicine that most physicians never see. Eventually, as you will see, I was given the chance to truly practice my art.

Chapter 1

Family Beginnings — It Started with a Bend in a River

I was born at the Gilmore Sanitarium on October 27, 1928, in Amory, Mississippi. Amory is located in the northeastern part of the state, approximately equidistant between Memphis, Tennessee, and Birmingham, Alabama, on the St. Louis-San Fransisco Railway, known as the Frisco. The distances are significant in that the main repair yards for the Frisco were located in Amory. There, the "round house" was located, where one could run large steam engines inside the building onto a large turntable and turn it toward any direction desired. The entire economy of the town was directly tied to the railroad. Everyone either worked directly or indirectly for the Frisco, as the place they worked depended on it for business. There was also a garment factory and a stave mill, which manufactured wooden staves for building barrels. This resulted in a town of lower middle-class families and a lot of poor people.

Since Amory is located very close to the Tombigbee River, there is good farmland located in the areas where the soil was enriched by the spring rains, causing the river to flood and deposit rich silt over the flat land. This is the reason it was called "bottom land." The building of flood control and navigational dams has effectively done away with this natural fertilization method. The farmers now have to use man-made fertilizer just like farmers everywhere. The farms located in these "bottom" areas planted mostly cotton and some corn and were fairly prosperous. Amory boasted of a population of five thousand people, though the actual population was more like three thousand. Everyone wanted to live in bigger towns in those days, even if it entailed fudging on the population figures. It was a good town to grow up in, because there were only a handful of rich people and an awful lot of not-so-rich people, so everyone got along fine. If any of the "rich" kids tried being snooty, they were quickly brought back to earth because there were no other "rich" kids to be snooty with.

The last time I was in Amory, it was pretty much the same as it was when I was growing up. The railroad ran through the middle of town in a northwestern to southeastern direction, and the town was spread in both directions along the tracks. On the northern side of the tracks was the business section of town and the main residential area. On the southern side of the tracks was the Styx, where the vast majority of the black people lived. This was segregation as it was practiced in those days, and no one thought anything of it.

The street one block off of the railroad was just commercial enterprises involved in the day-to-day activity of the railroad. Two blocks over from the railway station was Main Street, where pretty much all of the businesses were located. It was, and I think still is, three blocks long. It continues to the northeast as Highland Drive. It once was called Trace Road but, after they paved it, the powers that be changed it to a fancier name. After that, everyone still called it Trace Road. About one mile from the city limits, along this road on the right, is a red brick house where I lived and was reared until I was in the ninth grade. About fifty yards up the road on the right was my paternal grandparents' home. If one continues on this road, the small town of Smithville appears. Then it's on to Fulton, the county seat of Itawamba County, where my maternal kinfolk, the Boozers and the Wiyguls, lived.

My grandfather Bentley came to Amory while working for the Frisco railroad. He was a foreman on the water service. His duties included being in charge of a vital part of using steam as a source of power to run locomotives. This was the large elevated water tanks that one would see located along the tracks for mile after mile. These were strategically placed so the steam engine would be assured of having a sure source of water on board the locomotive. Steam was made by a very hot coal fire under the water boiler in the locomotive. The fire was maintained by the fireman who was located in the cab of the locomotive and stayed busy shoveling coal into the boiler throughout a trip. Since there was no electricity to run pumps for automatically filling the tanks, each water tank had employees who lived in shacks at each water tank along the railway line. It was a lonely life, usually without neighbors, and the pay was low, adding up to a hardscrabble existence. Their job was to use a gasoline-powered pump to transfer water from an adjacent well, thus keeping the huge water tanks full to the brim at all times. If there was a problem with the pump, the well, or the piping, it was my grandfather's job to get it fixed, either by himself or with a crew of men before the next train arrived.

One day, my grandfather got a message from one of the caretakers down the line that his gasoline water pump was not working properly. He caught the next train going in that direction, but by the time he got the pump repaired, the last train going back to Amory had already run. The caretaker told him that he could eat supper and breakfast with his family and sleep at his home. He readily accepted the invitation and, since he had worked hard all day long, he was ravenous by the time suppertime arrived. He sat down at the table, and they served him a heaping plate of collard greens and a large hunk of cornbread. Now if there was anything that my grandfather hated more than collard greens, I don't know what it was, unless it was boiled turnips. He used to growl, "Nobody could like turnips." He made the most of the cornbread that he could and decided that he would go to bed early. It was then that he discovered that the bed he was given to use was usually the bed for the family's old hound dog. During the mostly sleepless night, he fought with the hound dog as to which of them was going to sleep in that bed. Awakening sleepy and very hungry the next morning, he was looking forward to breakfast. He sat down at the table, and they served a heaping plate of cold collard greens and a large hunk of cold cornbread. Such was life in those days.

Before building a house of their own, the family lived in rental property in the downtown area. My father (Pap) had gotten a job as teller at the Security Bank of Amory, where he continued to work until the start of World War II. Jack, my youngest uncle, had not been born at this time and his brothers, Marshall and Rob, were in high school. Pap always loved cars and at one time owned a twelve-cylinder Studebaker sedan. He said it was a great car to drive but only got five miles to a gallon of gas. At this particular time he kept his new car parked in the family garage. Pap always was a late sleeper, and since he lived only a few blocks from his work, he took advantage of the situation to rise as close to 9:00 a.m. as possible.

Being enterprising young men and possessing a yen to drive Pap's new car also, Marshall and Rob would sneak out to the garage before school, push the car out of the garage down the street and crank it out of earshot of the sleeping owner. After a spin around town, they would drive the car back home; cut the engine off a safe distance from the house, and coast into the garage. Pap never realized what they were doing. In fact, he would brag about the car being so easy to start even on the coldest morning. All went well until one spring day when they were tooling down Trace Road with the top down. Upon cresting a small hill, they encountered a huge flock of Mr. Lantrip's white turkeys. There was no stopping or missing them, so they plowed into the midst. Turkeys went everywhere: to the sides, over the hood, and into the car. With the top down, turkeys and white feathers filled the the car. They drove on without stopping, I am sad to report.

They stopped down the road to wash the outside off and clean the turkey remains out of the car. Then they dutifully followed their usual procedure and coasted the car into the garage. All went well until Mr. Lantrip came into the bank later that morning and told Pap that he wanted to talk with him about killing a bunch of his turkeys. Pap said, "Mr. Lantrip, I haven't been out of town all morning. Try Buck Stockton; he has a car just like mine." It was years before his brothers told Pap the full story of what happened that day.

The Bentleys came to the southern and southwestern United States through a very circuitous route. It all began with a bend in a river. In olden England, a creek was known as a lay, and a bend in the river was known as a bent. So apparently, people who settled in a certain bend in the creek were called people from the bent lay. Somewhere and at some time, this was corrupted into Bentley. So much for the purity of gene strain in our ancestry, but we are related to the people who built the Bentley car.

In the years preceding the Revolutionary War, there were several brothers in our branch of the Bentley family. One of the oldest, Samuel, wanted to come to the colonies to live. The only other one who wanted to join him was the youngest son. Samuel then had to wait for his youngest brother to serve his apprenticeship as a shipwright. Since the youngest son had to be in a harbor town in order to practice his trade, he settled in Boston, Massachusetts, where he became good friends with a young silversmith named Paul Revere. For years my Dad told me this story, and I must say I just ignored it because my Dad was known to slightly embellish the truth. Years later while reading an article on Paul Revere in the journal *American Heritage*, I found a description of how the two men were close friends and the events leading up to his ride.

In the fever of the developing revolution and the need to warn the inhabitants of Lexington and Concord of the route the British were taking to put down the rebellious attitude there, the two friends and other revolutionaries hatched the famous plan. Riders were to be sent after lanterns were placed in the steeple of the Old North Church. The immortal words have been imbedded in every school attendee, "One if by land and two if by sea." Paul Revere was one of the riders, and he and Bentley made a plan to row across the Charles River to be in position to see the signals of lanterns hung in the steeple. From there, Revere would start his famous ride immortalized by Longfellow and warn the minutemen that the British were coming by land. Bentley would row the boat back across the river and dock it. On the night of the ride they gathered at the boat, but decided they needed something to muffle the oars in the oarlock. They walked a block or two over to Bentley's girlfriend's home and called up to her from below her balcony. After the pair explained their needs, a petticoat soon fluttered down "still warm from the body." This did a wonderful job of muffling the sounds of the oars, and the crossing was uneventful. The rest, as they say, is history.

The older brother apparently settled around Halifax, Virginia, sometime in the early 1700s. Unfortunately, I don't have the names of either of the original Bentley settlers. His son, Samuel, was born in Halifax, Virginia, and settled in Alexander, Virginia, where he was a farmer. He is reported to have grown foodstuffs for the revolutionary army after his uncle helped start the war. He had two sons who decided they wanted to go to the southern United States after the war in order to start their families.

The first brother, Samuel, Jr., stopped in Georgia, and all the Bentleys you see in Georgia and northern Alabama are scions of this man. It is important for my grandchildren to remember this fact, for I was in northern Alabama recently and the first thing my host asked me was, "Are you a descendent of Samuel?" I felt as if I belonged to some exclusive ritual society. (I don't really have enough family data, names, dates, siblings, etc., to form a meaningful family tree).

He had a son, Jeremiah Hall Bentley, who was born in Elbert, Georgia, in 1815. He, in turn, had a son, Richard Young Bentley, who was born in Forsyth, Georgia, in 1849. When a young man, Richard moved to Cass County, Texas, and established a homestead. He eventually married Mary Emma Clements in 1872. He was twenty-three at the time. My grandfather, Jeremiah, was born five years later.

A second brother, first name unknown, went into southern Louisiana to settle. He established a lumber business and apparently became very successful. There is a small town in south Louisiana, consisting of only a few stores, which is named for him. He was seemingly a character in the true sense of the word. He enjoyed going to the hotel in Alexandria to have his Sunday dinner. One Sunday, the head waiter would not let him into the dining room because he was not wearing a coat and tie. This so enraged the old man that he bought the hotel, and it is said that he enjoyed sitting on the veranda in his shirt sleeves. The Bentley Hotel still stands to this day.

My grandfather, whom I called Pa-Pa, was one of several brothers and sisters growing up in Texas. My granddaddy was a real live cowboy in his early life, and that is how he met my grandmother. He drove a herd of cattle into Cleburne, Texas, where she was living with her oldest sister. They apparently drove the cattle across some of her family land, and she went down to watch. There she said she saw "the handsomest man she had ever seen." Her name was Connie Ethel Cash, and yes, Johnny Cash was some distant cousin. She was a short little lady, about five feet tall, and one of the most cheerful people that I have ever known. Pa-Pa and Ma-Ma were married, and Pa-Pa subsequently went to work for the St. Louis-San Francisco railroad. They were stationed in Ashdown, Arkansas, where Herschel Paul, their first son, my dad (Pap), was born.

Ultimately they were transferred to Amory, Mississippi, and settled in to live there for the rest of their lives. They were existing peacefully when a strike, as I recall over wages and working conditions, was called against the Frisco railroad. The strike was broken, and my grandfather found himself in Amory with a baby boy, a wife, and no job. He met the problem head on and started his own business.

Since he had been working on the water service of the railroad, it was a natural transition to start his own plumbing and heating company. Ma-Ma had just borne fourth son, Jack Richard. Jack was twenty years younger than Herschel Paul. The second son was Marshall Clyde and the third, Robert Earl. All four sons and I, too, were required to learn the trade of plumbing and heating. In those days, all males were expected to learn a trade to insure that, if need be, one could always make a living working at that trade.

When I was born at the Gilmore Sanitarium, I was delivered by my maternal great uncle, Albert I. Boozer, M.D. He was Mama's "Uncle Albert," whom you will hear more about later. He and four brothers were born into a family of immigrants from Switzerland and were raised in Itawamba County, where his family tried to scratch out a living by farming those red clay hills. The name Boozer was apparently pronounced "Botzer" in their native country. It did not connote a family of hard drinkers. My grandfather James Presley, called Pres by his friends, was the oldest son, with four younger brothers, Albert, Elijah, Burley, and Joseph. My grandfather and great uncles, Albert, Elijah, and Burley, all wanted to be doctors. Uncle Joe was not so inclined, and he worked at odd jobs all of his life. He had one odd trait: he only liked the fat of meat and not the lean. Needless to say, he died at an early age of heart disease.

Since there was no money to send them to school, my grandfather, being the eldest, made the decision to go to work and use the money to send his three brothers to study medicine. The length of time required to earn a medical degree was not nearly so long as it is today, but still it took him a while to get them all graduated. To accomplish this, he became a carpenter and made his living as a house builder. My dad always said he could figure a job so close that the only scrap left over was sawdust. He eventually would build the house in Amory where we lived.

Uncle Albert started his practice in Amory, while Uncle Lige (Elijah) settled in Splunge, Mississippi, again up in the red clay hills. He had a truly rural general practice in which he made house calls on horseback with his medications and equipment in his saddle bags. Poor Uncle Burley died at the age of thirty-three after contracting tuberculosis from one of his patients.

My grandmother Boozer was born into the Wiygul clan in the Carolina community of Itawamba County, where her family also were farmers. Her name was Nancy Melverta Wiygul, and she had ambitions far beyond always living in the Carolina community. She went to college at Mississippi State College for Women when not many girls even thought about a college education. She said that during her first night at school, she was extremely scared, awfully lonesome, and terribly homesick. The dormitories were lit with natural gas lights, and when it got dark she didn't know how to light them. She had way too much pride to admit this, so she went to bed. One of her roommates came in and said something about not having the lights on, and she told her that she had a headache and was just lying quietly in the dark. All of her life she never had any patience with people who did not get all the education that they were capable of absorbing.

My maternal grandparents married and eventually settled in Shannon, Mississippi. They had four children: Uncle Riley Clinton, the oldest; then two boys who died in infancy, as was so common in those days; and my mother, Frankie Mae (all of his life, my grandfather called her Frank).

Uncle Riley was a dough boy in World War I and escaped unhurt. He was almost a savant in his learning ability. He could add a column of five figures as fast as I could add a column with one figure. He attended Ole Miss for one year, and he told me that he ended up with perfect scores in his math courses and Fs in all the rest of his subjects. He subsequently married a Shannon lady and they had one girl. Sadly, his wife died in childbirth, and he and his daughter, Mary Elizabeth (Beth) lived with his parents from that time on.

He was known for embellishing the truth, just like my dad. Unlike Dad, who always rubbed the back of his head when he lied, Uncle Riley would preface his whopper with, "Now this is the God's truth." He went into the concrete business and made a living during the Depression pouring concrete with a one-man concrete mixer, some wheelbarrows and Georgia buggies. . . . Later, he formed a partnership with his son-in-law, Henry Brevard, and they switched to the ready-mix concrete business; now B & B Ready-Mix plants are located all over northern Mississippi. Riley never married again, and as far as I know, never even dated anyone the rest of his life.

My grandparents were something like seventh cousins. For those living in a community with as small a population as Carolina it would very difficult to find someone who wasn't a very distant cousin. It was a constant source of concern for my mother, who was terrified that the marriage of cousins was going to unleash some rampant recessive gene that was going to make blithering idiots of either my brother Tom or me. Fortunately it did not, though some may argue with me about that.

One trait that has apparently been passed on from my Boozer grandparents is having a great compassion for the downtrodden. I will give you a classic example of this trait. After Riley was born, my grandfather heard about a boy who had lost his parents and was barely getting by hunting and fishing for his food. My grandfather talked with him about the opportunity of living with his family. The boy accepted his offer and lived with them for several years. My grandmother made sure the boy was well-educated and taught the proper etiquette necessary to navigate the social mores of the time. He eventually went into politics and was elected to the House of Representatives. He became powerful figure in the federal government, becoming chairman of several influential committees over the course of his forty-year tenure in the House. He was a strong backer of President Franklin Roosevelt and was a very conservative figure in Washington, D.C. His name was John Rankin. He said my grandparents never asked for a favor during the entire length of his political life.

As I said earlier, my grandfather was an accomplished carpenter and successfully made a living for his family building houses. This ended when he fell off a roof and broke his right hip and right wrist. After that, he always walked with a noticeable limp, and I'm told suffered with a stiff wrist. Together, these injuries kept him from pursuing construction work as a livelihood, and he quietly and confidently found other ways of making a living. This occurred during the Great Depression, which didn't make things any easier. He restarted in the town of Shannon, Mississippi, which is located about nine miles south of Tupelo.

In Shannon, he set up a gristmill. He ground corn not only into ordinary meal but also into a coarsely ground corn called "chops," which people used for chicken feed. Ordinarily, he would buy corn and grind it into meal for selling retail. I would help package it up in brown paper bags, carefully tied with string in peck quantities. To this day, I remember that a peck is twelve pounds. He then started a broom factory in the same building as his gristmill.

Subsequently, he would buy the Texaco gas station across the street. It had two pumps: one was electrically pumped and the other had a large lever, which when pushed back and forth, would pump the bright red gasoline into a round glass container sitting on top of the pump. This tank had gradient markings for each gallon. The customers would hand pump however many gallons they wanted, and then it was delivered by gravity. My cousin Beth and I agree that my grandfather really invented self-service at the gasoline pump. If you wanted gasoline from his pumps, you had to pump it yourself. I really liked to hand pump the gasoline, but he wouldn't let me. He said it would make people expect it when I wasn't there.

Grandfather was far too busy talking to his cronies to ever be interrupted. There was a long, low backless bench running along the front of the filling station front wall, and there each day various friends would drop in, sit, and whittle. It was interesting to me that they would bring their own block of wood for whittling. Apparently the men had their preferences of wood for carving. They would sit down and pull from their pockets a pocketknife and a block of wood. There was nothing special about the block of wood except it was easy whittling wood, such as cedar or fir. They would sit for hours, whittling away with razor-sharp pocketknives, just making paper thin coils of wood shavings. In this time they would thoroughly discuss the current weather and solve all the problems of the world.

Grandfather's building was located on one of the two paved streets of downtown Shannon. After the first block, the street turned to the left and then went another block. A right turn after the initial block led down an unpaved small hill. There, in the middle of the road, stood a large hand pump for the residents to get a cool drink of well water or to pump water for their animals. On Friday nights, the town government would set up a small movie screen at the base of this rise and show a film free of charge. These were usually oaters, movies about the frontier days of the Old West, or detective B-movies. The small hill now served as a movie theater with people sitting on the rise and the portable screen located at the bottom. The view of the screen was never obstructed by the person in front of you.

Alongside the town, one block away and down a small hill, the Baltimore and Ohio Railroad lines, or B&O, ran to the north and south. It had a small depot that was connected to the town of Shannon by two roads going down the slight hill. One was a paved road of downtown proper, and the other was an unpaved road that ran alongside my grandfather's building. Along this road was a blacksmith shop located directly across from the side door of the gristmill. The blacksmith was a hard-working man, and I would watch for hours as he made and put on horseshoes, wagon wheels and the like. Along this same road, farmers would travel wanting to get their corn ground into meal. As often as not, they would be riding bareback astride their old mule with a sack of corn thrown across its back. The corn would be weighed, and then it would either be ground for a fee, according to the weight, or ground for a fee based on some set percentage of the corn's weight. This was the barter system in use during the Depression.

Coincidental to all of this, my grandfather was also elected to be Justice of the Peace. His courtroom was the Gristmill and Broom factory building. Despite this being a building where they ordinarily ground meal and built brooms, when court was in session each business shut down, a nod to the solemnity of the occasion. The cases that came before the court were never serious legal problems, but usually included someone arrested for speeding by the newly formed Mississippi Highway Patrol. It could be two fellows arrested for fighting or being drunk in a dry state. It would be something that did not require an extensive knowledge of the law, but was easily handled by someone with common sense. If you were speeding, pay the fine. If you were fighting, explain your grievances. These were presented for judgment with all the solemnity of the great courts of the world. People were seated in straight-back oak chairs with woven cane bottoms, and the judge's bench was the same table on which I used to tie up my twelve-pound sacks of corn meal. At the end of the day, justice was served mainly by common horse sense.

Chapter 2

Family Settling — Making Homes in Hardscrabble Times

The Bentley family was well ensconced in Amory when I was born. All of the boys except Jack had graduated from high school. Pap had graduated from high school in 1918, and went to the University of Alabama for his freshman year. He was an outstanding athlete and played halfback on his high school and college football teams. This was the Alabama team that eventually went on to play in the first Alabama trip to the Rose Bowl. Pap wouldn't make this trip, however. Athletic scholarships were not so readily available in those days, and since there was no other source of money, his football playing days were over after his freshman year. However, that was not his only accomplishment while he was there. In addition to being a good athlete, he was an accomplished musician and played the trombone in the university band. While he was playing football, he was also the drum major of the Alabama marching band. This was before they were worth a million dollars. Still, I don't think that anyone has duplicated this feat since then.

Marshall Clyde was the next son chronologically. He played guard in football and was an excellent southpaw first baseman. He also was the placekicker for the Amory football team. He later attended Clarke Junior College and Ole Miss and, in addition to playing guard, was their placekicker in football as well as their first baseman in baseball. He went on to earn his master's in Education.

The year that Robert Earl was a senior in high school, Marshall kicked the field goal to win the game for Ole Miss over Mississippi State. The following year, Robert Earl got a scholarship to play guard on State's football team. When he reported for practice the first day, the coach said. "Bentley, huh. Are you kin to that Bentley that beat us last year?" Robert Earl stood tall and said, "No, sir."

Robert Earl did not get his scholarship renewed at the start of the next year because of a lack of funds, so he returned to Amory and decided to marry his high school sweetheart. Soon after the marriage, the school notified him that his scholarship was being renewed. However, married students weren't allowed to play on the football team, so his college career was over. He worked at several jobs then, but the one I remember the most was his driving the delivery truck for the Standard Oil Company. He would let me ride with him sometimes, and I would help him put the gasoline into the underground tanks. It was great fun as far as I was concerned. Eventually, he joined Pa-Pa in the plumbing business, and from then on it was known as J. M. Bentley and Son.

All of the Bentley boys tended toward being entrepreneurs. They were continually thinking up enterprises to make a little money. One of these was a movie theater in the area of town called The Styx. They rented a large building, put in some benches (no theater seats), and an elevated projector but were unable to install any form of heating. One night, Robert Earl said it was so cold that when he spilled some paste while putting up outside posters, it froze before it could stop running. Inside, a "cowboy show" was being shown, and the hero was being chased by the bad guys. As so often happened in these epics, the hero came upon a cliff with no escape path evident on either side. Fortunately, as he looked down, there was a river down at the bottom of the cliff, as there always was. As the hero was sitting astride his horse contemplating his next move, a voice from the audience intoned, "He ain't gonna jump, and it's too cold."

Jack was still in high school when I was just a small boy. Since we were in different buildings, I never saw him at school. On Friday nights during the football season, we always went to the home games and watched him play center on the football team. After graduating from high school, he began to work as a plumber with Pa-Pa and Rob.

After the start of World War II, there were construction jobs available everywhere in America for skilled laborers. Jack and Rob moved to Anniston, Alabama, and began working at Fort McClellan on a defense project. Because Jack was so young, the plumber's union was hesitant to put him to work as a journeyman plumber. They gave him a practical examination at the workplace. He passed the test with ease and became a journeyman plumber at the tender age of seventeen. No one in the family thought too much about this accomplishment because he had been doing plumbing for at least eight years. Later, they would move to Huntsville to help build the Redstone Arsenal. This was converted after the War to building Saturn rockets that took astronauts to the moon. Soon his time came up in the draft, so he joined the Army Air Corp. He piloted bombers, and after the War, he married Blanche Hoffman, whom he met while stationed in Nebraska. Of course, he was eligible for the G.I. Bill, so he reasoned that if he were going to college, why not try for the best? He applied to Harvard University and was accepted. He stayed there long enough to earn a bachelor's degree in engineering and a master's degree in business. He was one of those chosen when Henry Ford II hired a large number of MBAs from Harvard to help get automobile production cranked up again at Ford Motor Company.

My family lived about a mile from the city limits in a two-bedroom, dark-red brick house that was built by Grandfather Boozer. It was the first house in the community to feature the high-pitched roofs so common during the 1920s. I remember people driving by and stopping in the road to look at it. I don't know whether they approved of it or not. I have very few memories of living there until my brother, Tom, was born. I distinctly remember being very upset when he messed up his diapers for the first time. I became aware that little brothers did such things and didn't use the bathroom like the rest of us. I was truly incensed to have such a dumb brother.

It was about this time that Pap became interested in woodworking. He began to stop by Mr. Hathcote's woodworking shop for lessons. Mr. Hathcote was an excellent craftsman and an excellent choice for a mentor. He was no lover of machines, preferring to do most delicate work by hand. Thus my dad learned the intricacies of hand crafting from an expert. Later he would convey this knowledge to my brother Tom and me.

Dad began to crave a shop of his own. There was a small enclosed back porch leading from the kitchen to the backyard, and Pap decided he would make this approximately five-by-seven foot area into his first workshop. He built himself a workbench the length of the room and constructed it so that pieces of wood placed in the vise could extend into the kitchen. Many mornings Mama would walk into the kitchen after Pap had been using the plane the previous evening and face a huge pile of shavings. She apparently handled this with her usual good humor because I don't remember her complaining. Pap also kept paint and things like varnish remover stored there. This led to one of my brother's many escapades as the family imp, which I will share later.

Tom was born with a sadistic sense of humor that he inherited from our Grandfather Boozer. Our grandfather was one of the kindest and most compassionate individuals ever known. This is evidenced by him having literally saved John Rankin off a creek bank, an episode in his life told earlier. However, Grandpa Boozer loved to play practical jokes, and sometimes they could border on the cruel.

I recall one of these jokes when Tom was about five or six years old. We were visiting the grandparents for the weekend, and we were all sitting around the wood-burning stove in the second bedroom. Tom began to fuss and cry that he wanted to go outside by himself. It was after dark, and we weren't allowed to go outside alone after dark. Finally Grandpa said it would be all right for him to go. Tom quickly went into the long center hall and turned left into the foyer and out the front door. Unbeknownst to Tom, Grandpa followed him down the hall, and as soon as Tom closed the front door, he cut off the light in the foyer. The entire front of the house went into pitch black darkness. Immediately, the front door crashed open with Tom at top speed. He tripped and fell but didn't take time to right himself. He just started crawling at full speed, down the dark center hall and into the bedroom. He was followed by Grandpa laughing so hard he couldn't speak. He just stood there with his mouth open as if laughing, but no sound was heard. He had to lean against the wall to keep from falling. Soon he got himself under control and was able to talk. This was his idea of humor and Tom inherited it, unchanged.

The very first such episode I recall was when Tom was about two years of age. He had just been given a tin horn to play with, and he was running around tooting on this thing. It was time for Pap to wake up and get ready for work, so Mama told him. "Tom, go in and wake Daddy with your new horn." With that, he toddled off to the bedroom and hit Pap in the head with his new horn. Pap jumped out of bed and yelled, "Good God, Tom. You've killed me! " As usual,

Mama tried hard not to snicker but she lost the battle. At least it got Pap out of bed.

Several months later, Pap was dressing one morning and was having trouble getting one shoe on. He could get his toes in, but then he would hit some sort of obstruction. He finally picked up the shoe and looked inside. There was a mousetrap all set, but fortunately for Tom—as it probably saved him from a spanking—the lever that crashes down on a mouse's neck (or unsuspecting toes) was hung up on the tongue of the shoe.

Mama always raised a pig every year. Her parents would raise a calf, and Mama would provide the pork for the combined families. Tom would make a pet of the pig every year, and every year the pig would "get out of the pen" and never be seen again. This always occurred in the fall, when it became chilly and was referred to as "hog-killing time." Tom never did catch on to what was really happening to his pet pigs. This one particular year, Mama was just breaking even on the cost of raising the pig and the cost of just buying the meat. Pa-pa used to say, "We eat everything but the oink." Mama had rendered all the fat into five gallons of lard, and she figured that this was pure profit. She put the five gallons of lard in the kitchen and left, feeling pretty good about the whole thing. When she returned, she found that Tom had gotten the varnish remover out of Pap's stash on the back porch. He was apparently emulating Mama's cooking procedures and was standing there pouring and stirring varnish remover into her carefully-rendered lard. The lard was ruined, and the pig's demise didn't save money. We as a family didn't discuss raising pigs any more for the rest of the year.

The epitome of his youthful escapades has become an integral part of family lore. Our home in Amory had beautiful, oak hardwood floors that I am sure that Grandfather Boozer had labored over long and hard. These were Mama's pride and joy, and she kept them spotless and highly polished. Thus, they made a perfect place to run and slide in our socks. One afternoon Mama had gone up to visit my grandmother; she left Tom and some friend of his and our first cousin Jean to play at the house. The children were old enough to be left alone, but I don't remember their exact ages. They were enjoying themselves immensely, sliding on the hardwood floors in their socks, when Tom got one of his devilish ideas.

He decided could make a really keen skating rink if he dusted the floor with flour, make the hardwood surface even slicker. In those days, people bought their flour in twenty-four-pound sacks made of gingham material that could be used to make a dress for a small girl. It was common to see girls at school wearing dresses made of sack cloth. So Tom got out the flour sifter and proceeded to sift flour over all the floors and furniture in the house. His plan worked wonderfully well and provided unmatched floor skating.

Then Jean got a pang of conscious and decided that she was going to tell Aunt Frankie what was going on. Tom got worried about the flour and the resulting mess, so he took on the daunting task of cleaning it up. He found the vacuum cleaner hose and started pouring water around to wash up the white mess. Of course, this turned the flour into a sticky, gooey paste. At the height of this folly, Mama came through the door. Tom said she got really mad extremely fast. She gave him a good spanking then began dragging him by the arm into the various rooms of the house. As she would enter each room and see the mess, she would reach down and give him another swat. There were seven rooms. It was a long time before Mama could see any humor in the escapade, if she ever did.

Many years later, Tom bought himself a sailboat. This was after Mama and Pap had moved to live on Mobile Bay just below Point Clear, Alabama. He got a great buy, he said, but apparently he failed to notice the massive amount of rot that had consumed a large part of the boat, including some vital structures such as ribs and siding. Undaunted, he and Pap toiled over the boat for many months, and they finally reached the goal of seaworthiness. Tom began to sail and one day offered to take our cousin Henry Brevard on a little sailing jaunt. They were out in the Bay, far enough that the shoreline was only a gray indistinct haze on the horizon, when Henry turned to Tom and said, "Tom, where did you learn to sail?" Tom replied, "I bought me a book, but I haven't finished it yet."

Chapter 3

Childhood in an Era of Kindness and Gentleness

As I said before, we lived out on Highland Drive about one mile from town. Pa-pa lived on some land next to ours that he had bought after establishing his new business. When he first built his home, there was no electricity available in that area. He built the house with "indoor" plumbing and radiator heat, all of which required running water. There were no water mains built out that way, and he solved the problem by digging a shallow well. The water table in that area was only fifteen or so feet below the surface.

He then put his railroad experience to use. In the backyard, he built a huge cypress water tank, just like those used by the railroad. He then installed a gasoline water pump in the well and ran a pipe from the pump to the water tank. Each day or so he would crank the pump and refill the tank. The tank was suspended in the air on large cypress posts sitting on top of huge, solid-concrete blocks, and the tank was high enough to furnish good water pressure in the house—entirely by gravity. In fact, he ran a large water pipe from the tank to our home, about fifty yards down the road that also furnished our house with water. Pap eventually dug an underground fruit cellar that also contained a shallow well and electric pump.

Northeast Mississippi was the first area in the country to receive TVA electricity. This occurred before I have any memory. Our house was wired for electricity when it was built, but Pa-pa's had not been.

Like many homes, it had wiring installed afterward. These homes usually started out with a long electrical cord, with a bare light bulb shining brightly, hanging from the center of the room. The bulb was turned off or on with a switch on a long cord or light chain hanging down from the light socket.

Ma-ma, my paternal grandmother, had a 1938 Ford sedan that carried her around town. She was very short, so much so that she had to peer through the steering wheel to see where she was going. She never went anywhere without her hat and white gloves. The hat would raise her profile enough so that people could see that there was someone behind the wheel and that the car was not wheeling driverless down the road. It was far better than another elderly gentleman in town, who was such a bad driver that all the children were instructed that if we saw his car, we were to get as far away as we could from the street.

At any rate, Ma-ma had a hard time seeing the entrance to a driveway because of her low position, and she had a tendency to swerve to the middle of the road so she could see to turn into the entrance. One day she arrived home, swerved out to the left, and turned right to go into her driveway. Suddenly, a car that had been following her slammed into the passenger's side of her car. The driver got out of his car and exclaimed, "Lady, you didn't signal!" Ma-ma replied, "Well, I've been living here for forty years."

Living out there was idyllic for a young boy. About one hundred yards down the road toward town lived the Rogers family. The patriarch of this enclave was "Brother" Rogers, an itinerant Baptist preacher. He lived there with his wife, whom we called "Mama" Rogers; their son, Joel Berry, and two daughters, Lucille and Camille. Sitting in a grove of large oak and pecan trees, the old one-story sprawling house featured large porches on the front and down one side.

As was common with these homes surrounded by large trees with dense foliage, it was so shady that grass would not grow, and the yards would be barren with the clay soil packed hard. The residents kept them swept daily with brooms made of stick bundles. The house was surrounded by outbuildings, which housed machinery and necessary equipment needed to operate an active farm. Also, these farms usually had a barn with a large hayloft and stalls for feeding and milking the cows.

Like every country house in those days, there was a drilled

artesian well with a large pipe coming out of the ground topped by a large pipe fitting which made a ninety-degree turn. This resulted in a short pipe running parallel to the ground. The end of this pipe was cut off on a slant, making it easier for someone to drink. The amount of water that flowed was dependent on the size of pipe with which the well was drilled. If you had a large pipe you had a large spout of water coming out, or if it was a relatively small pipe, then you had a much smaller flow of water. These ran constantly and thus were termed ever-flowing wells. The water coming from these wells was cold as ice water and had a peculiar taste, the likes of which I have never tasted since. It obviously contained a great deal of iron because the ditches that carried the runoff water from the well were coated with iron oxide, which glowed reddish brown on the sides of the canal and surrounding vegetation. Iron deficiency anemia was definitely not a common malady in this countryside.

Because of the cold water, the populace used these wells to keep their milk cold. The water spewing out of the well spouts emptied into a "milk trough." These troughs were made of either lumber or concrete and were large enough to hold several gallon buckets or milk cans, with the water high enough to cover all the sides of the vessels. The water ran constantly and kept the milk cold and unspoiled. The Rogers' milk shed was large, since they had several cows. What really fascinated me about it was a Confederate calvary sword which stayed in there. It was not on display, but simply was kept there. It belonged to a relative who rode with General Nathan B. Forrest, who was not only Forrest Gump's namesake, but also had the military strategy of "getting there firstest with the mostest." My favorite spot in this area was a shallow-well pitcher pump that was located in the backyard under the large trees. Children could be hot, sweaty, and thirsty from hard playing and run up to this pump, give it a few pumps, and drink their fill of cold, clear (normal) water.

Neither of the Rogers' daughters was married. Lucille taught English at the high school and taught Rob in the tenth grade. He loved to tell the story of a disgruntled classmate who approached Lucille after having a test returned with a "0" awarded as a grade. He stood at her desk and said, "Miss Rogers, I don't believe I deserved a '0' on this test."

She looked up at him and said, "I know you didn't, but that was as low as I could give you."

Also on this property, and closer to our house, was a small

stucco white house built in the Spanish style. Here lived the next oldest Rogers son, Halbert (the oldest, Daniel, had previously moved to Texas). No one knew him by that name, however, and he was affectionately known everywhere as "Zook." They had a son, Halbert, Jr., who was better known as Hal and was my best friend growing up. He was a year older than I, and as we grew older and into high school, where age matters, we tended to grow apart. However, before we grew older, we were thicker than thieves.

There was a large field between his house and mine where Jo-Ber usually planted cotton. Of course, when the cotton plants grew tall, they afforded a serious impediment to our getting from one house to the other without having to walk out to the road and down the right-of-way. This required more energy than we wanted to expend, so every spring when the cotton began to come up, we would start a path by walking across the field. We stomped down cotton plants selectively, so there was a straight path across the field where no cotton grew. Jo-Ber never complained to us about our path-making.

Jo-Ber was the farmer of the Rogers family and planted large fields of cotton and corn on both sides of the highway. Behind the main house stretched a large pasture that ended on a tiny stream called Burkett's Creek. In my childhood, this seemed like a large body of water, but the reality was an adult could step across in most places. There was one wide area that must have been six- or eight-feet in width but was very shallow. Hal and I solved this problem by taking burlap bags, filling them with dirt, and piling them at the narrow exit of this little pond. Miraculously, the pond increased in depth until it was really deep. It would be up to your waist if you stood up, and up to your neck if you squatted down.

Nevertheless, it allowed us to tie a rope to a lower limb of an overhanging oak tree growing on the edge of our swimming hole. We spent hours swinging out over the water and letting go, splashing into our "deep" water. The creek had eroded underneath the roots of the oak and left a hollow there with roots hanging down. It served to make this a scary-looking place. Every once in a while, we would find an old water moccasin under there and would have to scare him out of our swimming hole. It really was not deep enough for swimming,

Occasionally our folks would carry us over to Okolona, Mississippi, about fifteen miles away, where they had a municipal pool with deep water and high and low diving boards. This was a real treat, and many times it would end with a picnic in the adjacent park. Ah, life was sweet.

It usually snowed two or three times a year. When it did, everyone made snow ice cream, which consisted of a glass full of clean snow, a teaspoon of vanilla flavoring, sugar to taste, and fresh milk poured to the brim of the glass. This truly was the nectar of the gods. After this, everyone would congregate across the road at Ross's Hill for a sledding experience. Mrs. Ross was a widower who lived across the highway from my grandparents. She lived there alone, though she had a son, Bill, who saw to her needs and comfort. She owned several acres of land there and kept the usual food-producing animals, such as chickens, etc.

In the back of her house was a fairly high hill with a gentle slope that ended in a flat area. This allowed sufficient space to let one's sledding momentum die down before reaching the tree line along a little stream that meandered across the back of her property. She seemed to thoroughly enjoy all the people coming over and sliding down her snow-covered hill. People came with all sorts of things, such as garbage can lids and boxes, to slide on. We and others had homemade sleds made with two-by-four inch lumber planks and connected by one-inch planks nailed across them. The two-by-fours were cut on a slant in the front to serve as sled runners. They served the purpose wonderfully well, and many happy hours were spent in these pursuits. Leather gloves were not available to us children in those days, and we all had gloves made of some sort of cloth. They worked fairly well until the cloth eventually got wet from the snow. Then fingers turned to ice cubes, and the owner of the damp gloves had to ponder whether to stop and go warm his or her hands and gloves or risk frostbite. We had the same problem when we built snowmen. I don't really remember anyone developing frostbite.

Located next to Mrs. Ross were the Caldwells. Their driveway struck the highway across the road, midway between our driveway and my grandparents'. Papa Caldwell had farmed their land until he became so crippled with arthritis that he could no longer do physical work. He was a stocky man who was always jovial and extremely gracious. He could maneuver very slowly with the aid of two canes. He had a large, fluid-filled sac about the size of a football located on the anterior right side of his neck. This was non-tender and obviously very soft. It was probably a lymphangioma that today would just be removed, but this was not available in those days.

He usually spent his days sitting on the front porch in the summer and in front of a fireplace with a large log fire blazing in the winter. He loved to play dominoes and almost always had some visiting soul to play double-twelve dominoes with. It was always cut-throat competition. Mama Caldwell kept the family fed, the house clean, and did all the necessary chores to run a household with chickens, cows, pigs, and geese. Consequently, I only remember her looking as if she were dog-tired. She was a short, stocky woman who was always pleasant, but never joked or kidded. Life was far too realistic and somber for her to be that way. When Papa Caldwell died many years later, she came to live with Mama and Pap in Fairhope instead. This was at Mama's insistence. History does have a habit of repeating itself.

The Caldwells had a fairly large farm and, after no longer being able to farm it, they sold the farming rights to the Rogers and lived off this income. The house was one of the typical sprawling, white-clapboard homes. The porch spread across the entire length of the front of the house and had a large swing at one end, chairs scattered around, and a card table for the domino contests. The front yard contained the usual large oak trees with the barren front yard, carefully swept with stick brooms. Behind the house were the pig pens, hen houses, and the barn.

The barn always had straw on the floor from spillage occurring while the cows were fed, and it was there that the geese chose to lay their eggs. Geese always lay their eggs in a hastily made straw nest and then carefully cover them up, so the nest is not different than its surroundings. It was great fun for me to help Mama Caldwell find these so-carefully-hidden eggs. Every so often, when we found several of the huge eggs, she would award my help by giving me an egg to take home. I would very proudly present the egg to my mother, who would cook it for me. One goose egg would equal three or four hen eggs.

Behind this house was a place of sheer enjoyment for young boys like Hal and myself. There was a large gravel pit where they had dug out large amounts of river gravel that had been deposited there eons before, leaving a place with steep cliffs, reedy ponds, and innumerable rocks to throw and to serve as ammunition for our slingshots. On the other side of the house to the back and down the hill, there was a small, clear, freely running spring. The spring itself was about three feet in diameter and probably two feet deep. The runoff from the spring ran on down the hill and ended in a pond about an acre in size.

Papa Caldwell had built an earthen dam that formed the pond. It was constantly being fed from the spring, and it flowed out through a sluiceway at the other end. It was stocked with bass and bream, but for the life of me, I can't remember catching any fish there. It was well stocked with other creatures that were not intentionally placed there, such as water moccasins. One or two could always be seen swimming across the pond with their heads held high above the water. Their presence never intimidated us from going down to the pond, but we were always wary of them. More than once we got close to one, realizing it luckily enough before it spotted us, but we never came close to being bitten. We played near the water but never tried to go swimming in it, although more than once we tried to build a raft, à la Tom Sawyer. We never succeeded, however, in getting one that would truly float and support our combined weights at the same time.

Back up the path to the house was a large wild-plum thicket bearing both yellow and red succulent plums. In the fall, when these plums became ripe, we would crawl under the canopy of plum bushes, sit down, and eat those sweet, juicy morsels until we were stuffed. When I remember that little path in the weeds and grass going down to the spring, it always reminds me of one of Pa-pa's Pat and Mike jokes.

Pa-pa always had Pat and Mike stories to fit every occasion. One day, Pat and Mike were walking down this hot, dusty road, and they became very thirsty. In a move that was not unusual in those days, they approached the front door of a house along the road. Pat walked up, and, hat in hand, he knocked on the front door. When a lady came to the door, he explained their need for a cool drink of water. She replied, "Of course, just go down the path to the spring and you will find a dipper there. Drink all that you want." Pat put his hat back on and started walking down the path. Shortly, he met a turtle walking toward the house. Now, Pat had never seen a turtle before, and he studied it a few minutes and abruptly turned on his heel and walked back to the house. He knocked on the door, and when the lady of the house again answered, he announced, "Ma'am, I hate to have to tell you that your spring has evidently gone dry. I met your dipper walking back to the house." All of his tales weren't always that funny.

Along the hillside by the spring there was small forest of red cedar trees. Red cedar trees were well suited to growing in the environs of that part of Mississippi, and they grew in abundance along fence rows and anywhere that wasn't cultivated. Sawmills would cut the large ones, and the planks were commonly used for lining closets or making chests for storing things that otherwise might be eaten by moths. No matter how old the lumber became, it never lost its aromatic quality. These young trees also had another thing they were perfect for—they made Christmas trees.

When I got old enough, it was my job to cross the road, go behind the Caldwell house, find the perfect tree, saw it down, and drag it home. I would make a wooden stand, attach it, and set it up in the living room. We would all participate in the decorating of the tree. Santa could always be depended on to bring a crate of oranges that got put under the tree and into our stockings. This was usually our taste of citrus for the year. Stores could only get citrus fruit shipped in during the growing and ripening seasons of Florida. Citrus was just not shipped across the country or up from South America to small Mississippi towns. Fortunately for us, this corresponded to the Christmas season. If there was enough money for a big Christmas, then we got a crate of tangerines also.

Now, that was really a treat and one that I, in particular, really enjoyed. I liked tangerines more than I liked oranges. Another thing would be some fireworks. The amount and variety might vary according to the money available, but there were always Roman candles, sparklers, and sometimes sky-rockets. On Christmas night, we would always have a fireworks show. On one occasion in the afternoon of Christmas day, Tom got into the stash of Roman candles, took one out, stuck the fuse end into the space heater, and soon had brightly-colored fireballs bouncing off the walls and curtains of the dining room. It was actually a funny sight with Mama chasing Tom to get the Roman candle, and Tom laughing, running, and firing away. The candle held only ten shots, and fortunately there were no fires ignited. With no damage being done, and taking Tom's young age at the time into account, no punishment was instituted.

When I would go over to that hillside and look down on that pond, it always reminded me of another of Pa-pa's Pat and Mike stories. One day, Pat and Mike were out in a boat doing a little fishing. They were a rather far distance from the shore, but neither of them were worried about that. Pat stood up in the boat and did a little stretching. When he did, the boat flipped, and they both found themselves treading water.

Pat says to Mike, "Mike, I don't know how to pray, but you better say a prayer."

Mike says to Pat, "Pat, I don't know how to pray either."

Pat says, "Then let's take up collection; we've got to do something religious."

In my younger years before starting school, Pap got into the chicken business along with Mr. Staub, who also owned a hardware store in Amory. They weren't raising chickens for eggs or eating, but they were raising and selling show chickens. They raised Barred Rock chickens because they were both good layers of eggs and also big enough to be good meat producers as well. They kept very precise records of the genetic makeup of the producers of the eggs, and then they would sell the eggs to someone who wanted to start a flock of chickens for a commercial business.

Barred Rock chickens are black with white speckles. The feathers are black, with the base of the feathers being white in a semi-lunar configuration. This left a black chicken spotted all over with small, white semicircular speckles. Pap and Mr. Staub would take chickens in wire cages to fairs all over the South and Midwest. Before taking them, he would groom them meticulously and even polish their feathers with a silk cloth. He collected so many blue ribbons that Mama made a bedspread out of some of them. In addition, he had red ribbons for second place and white ribbons for third place. These weren't given any place of honor but were stuck in a drawer someplace.

One year, one of his roosters was named the National Champion at a fair in Chicago. He was then able to sell eggs fertilized by this old fellow for a dollar apiece. That was a lot of money in those days. In fact, it was a day's wage for a lot of people with day-labor jobs. "Another day, another dollar—a million days, a million dollars," was a common saying in those days. Pap would pack the eggs for shipment in our house. He would carefully wash and clean every egg, polish them with a silk cloth, and individually wrap them in newspaper. Then he would embed each egg in a bed of excelsior. I don't remember him ever telling us that some eggs were broken in shipment.

Now, that old rooster was a really mean fowl. He ruled the chicken yard with an iron hand, and he didn't want anything or anybody else in the yard without his blessing. The trouble was that his chicken yard and our backyard were one and the same. He was a huge bird, and he had spurs about two inches long. If he didn't want you around, he would run at you with his wings flapping and propel himself at you with both feet well out front, so as to get you good with those spurs. One day he decided that he didn't want me around in my own backyard, and he started to chase me. I reached down and grabbed a corn cob and flung it with all my might. It cracked him right on the side of his head. He fell to the ground as if he had been shot and began flapping his wings like chickens do when you wring their necks. I was scared to death that I had killed Pap's champion rooster. To my great relief, he got up few seconds later and wobbled off to his harem. From then on, we gave each other a wide berth.

My job with the chickens was burial detail. Whenever a chicken died, it was my job to bury it. My method was to take a posthole digger and make a posthole large enough to contain the carcass of the departed chicken. Then with a shovel I would scoop up the bird and stuff it into the posthole head first. It had to be deep enough so that the feet would not be sticking out. That definitely was bad form. Then a little dirt thrown in the hole, tamped down with my bare foot, and the job was done. It wasn't a bad job, until we found a chicken that had been dead for several days and reeked to high heaven. The entire process had to be done while breathing in only a few times, and then in small gasps. I think this prepared me for the odors of the dissecting lab in gross anatomy, or the autopsy room later in medical school. At least those smells of corpses in anatomy lab and the autopsy room didn't bother me very much; I had worked with something that smelled much worse.

By the time that Pap got out of the chicken trade, he had gone from having one gray stucco henhouse to three. The newer buildings were very large and contained a great deal of square footage under a roof. Eventually they would be changed to lumber storage, including areas where the lumber could be stacked for air drying, and it would stay there undisturbed for a year or more. In the interim, Pap had graduated from the back porch to building the first of three "garages" that would be his workshops. He now went into the business of building furniture and kitchen cabinets, and repairing and restoring furniture.

The "garage" began to grow like a dirt dauber's nest. First, there was a larger building erected across the back of the original building.

This was heated in the winter by a potbellied stove that burned shop wood scraps for fuel. At times, when it was exceptionally cold outside, the stove would glow red from the fierce fire glowing in her bowels. I don't think it ever occurred to anyone that this was a fire hazard. Soon another building was added behind the first addition. This was the spray area, and it was large enough to hold a car. With the hiring of some more workers, this became a new part of the business. Here was where I began to learn the woodworking business. I started out making wooden rubber guns, graduated to making wooden swords, and on to making benches for our tennis court.

In my young years, Pap had severe headaches that would literally incapacitate him. During one of these bouts, Mama called Uncle Albert and told him about the headaches and that she had given Pap sixteen aspirin tablets. His reply was, "Well, that's a God's plenty." She was always calling Uncle Albert about one thing or another, and I am sure that she worried him to death. However, being the extremely patient man that he was, he never complained to my knowledge. Another time she called him and said, "Uncle Albert, I have broken my thermometer." He replied, "Well for God's sake don't buy another one."

When the headaches continued, Mama convinced Pap to go and see Uncle Albert. After listening to his complaints and examining him, he declared, "You know, Herschel, I have been taking care of farmers in this area who consistently work extremely hard from daylight to dark. Yet I have never seen one who complained about headaches. I believe that you are not getting enough exercise. You need to find some sort of exercise that you enjoy and do it."

Pap talked it over with Joel Rogers, and they decided to take up tennis. They first built a clay court right next to the Rogers' house. Later, they would build two courts on a piece of the Rogers' land that was on hard clay ground, up a slight hill beyond Burkett's Creek. They began to play regularly, and soon many other people began to make the trip out to the tennis courts. They began to enter tournaments, both in doubles and singles. Pap was a very good athlete, and he began to win in tournaments throughout the South. One year, he was even Southern Champ. Incidentally, his headaches disappeared. Hal and I would go up to the courts and would be ball boys. Our job was to kneel down by the net at the net post. Then, whenever a first service ball hit the net, we would run across, pick up the tennis ball, and run to the other side and kneel there. We also had to run down balls hit over the backstops.

Road conditions going to the two courts became hazardous. The road surface was only graded red clay, which became very slippery when wet. In addition, the ditches on each side of the road began to erode from rainwater which left less road surface and markedly deeper ditches. It was decided that a new court needed to be built in a different location. For this, they turned to Pa-pa. Pa-pa mowed his yard up to a row of Lombardy poplar trees along the side yard. Beyond this was a small pecan orchard. They decided that this was the perfect place to put in a new court. I don't know how they convinced him of this, but with the provision that his garden, which backed up to this land, would not get trampled, he agreed.

The barbed-wire fence that surrounded the pecan orchard was moved over the required amount, and tall backstops, made from whitewashed telephone poles, were set up so that balls would seldom find their way into the garden. Both ends were covered with chicken wire so the area was secured from wandering balls. Then truckloads of dark red clay were brought in and dumped over the tennis court area. It was Hal's and my job to spread the clay over the area of the new court. We would load clay into a wheelbarrow, push it over to the area that needed it, and we would dump it. While one wheeled the clay, the other would spread it.

Until you've done this, you have no idea how a little wheelbarrow full of clay changes a pile of clay carried away from a momentous pile of dirt. Eventually the clay was spread, the court was made perfectly level, the dimensions were laid out, and the net posts were cemented in place. We were ready to play tennis, and play we did. We played from daylight 'til dark, and were inconsolable when it rained. People would come from all over to play, and thus was the need for benches to be made.

Hal and I got good enough that we were entering tournaments held in town. We were only in junior high school so no one expected us to win against the adults, but we usually advanced several brackets before being eliminated. I'm sure the adults that we beat were chagrined about being beaten by a couple of junior high school kids, but we did, after all, spend every waking minute on the court. I continued to play into my college days, but I never was as good as my old man. I didn't play anymore until my son, John, wanted to be on the tennis team in high school. I came out of retirement to let him practice and beat up on me. I haven't played since.

The Amory school system was unusual. The public elementary, junior high school, and the high school were private schools. There was an academic board made up of educational personnel as well as private citizens. I don't know how the finances were arranged with the state, but the school board held autonomy. The teachers had to maintain continuing education courses, and the failure rate of their students was carefully scrutinized. Of course, in this small town, the teachers and parents were pretty sure to know each other.

There were two classes for every grade, labeled A or B, which denoted at what level the classes were taught. If one were in an A class, it meant that your studies were pushed faster and more in depth. I don't remember any stigma that was attached to being put in the B class. Everyone looked at it as a normal thing, with those students needing a little more time to learn. I can remember studying Shakespeare in depth in the seventh grade. Most of the teachers had been teaching there for long periods of time, and usually had taught our parents and relatives. In fact, the principal of the junior and high school was the same lady who was there for my dad.

I'm sure that she thought of me as the son of that boy who, on his motorcycle, entered one side door of the first floor, rode the width of the building, and out the opposing side door. Pap was accompanied on this excursion by Dudley Rowan, riding behind him on the seat. Dudley (better known as "custard head") would go on to be Mayor of Amory for many years and own a first-class hardware store. His youngest daughter, Rose, was my first date going to a Cub Scout banquet in the seventh grade. She would later marry my best friend.

I came from a musical family. My mother played the piano, sang alto, and she was very active in the Amory Music Club. Pap was musically inclined also. I have already alluded to his playing trombone while attending the University of Alabama. After settling down in Amory, he continued to play his trombone. He played in an orchestra called King Coyle's Own, and apparently they were kept busy playing for dances.

He told me about an episode involving a new music selection for the band. They belonged to some type of club with music publishers that resembled the Book Club. When they had new songs, they would send them sheet music, with words and music for their perusal. They got one of a new song by Irving Berlin, and after playing it and reading the lyrics, they decided this one wasn't going anywhere and they let it go. It turned out to be one of the biggest hits ever written. It was named *My Blue Heaven.* "Just Molly and me, and baby makes three, in my blue heaven." In addition, Pap played in the American Legion Band that was headquartered in Tupelo, Mississippi. This was a very active organization, and they traveled to a lot of cities to play, including being invited one time to be in a parade in New York City. Everyone was dutifully impressed. They wore military uniforms with bright, shiny buttons, and their hats were like the steel helmets the dough boys wore in World War I, except they were made of bright, shiny brass.

In addition to our music heritage, the Bentleys were very involved with athletics. All played football, baseball, and softball. One summer, when I was a little shaver, Pa-pa sponsored a softball team for the local softball league. All four of his sons played, and Joel Rogers was the pitcher. They were called "The Plumbers," and wore light blue shirts, with the name "Plumbers" sewn on the back. The letters were cut out of red felt by my Uncle Jack and sewn on by Ma-ma.

With all the family history of playing football, everyone expected me to play football. I started out playing in seventh grade, and because of my size, started out as a guard. This changed after a while, and I was put in the backfield, playing fullback. I was happy with that situation, but I found out that there were two different weight limits to be met before playing. The first was 110 lbs., and the second was 125 lbs. There was no way that I was ever going to make 110 lbs., so I was limited to playing with the "big boys." I only remember playing in one game, and don't even remember our opponent. I just remember taking a handoff on a reverse, and I came around left end like a runaway freight train. I went about five yards before this guy tackled me from behind, and I landed on my head. I went one way, and the ball went another. After the game, Pap told me I was carrying the ball in my left arm like it was a loaf of bread.

I played football all my grade school years. I finally was permanently placed in the backfield playing quarterback and halfback on offense, and linebacker on defense. We weren't sissies in those days; you stayed out there every play unless someone carried you off the field. Harrumph! I made All Conference my senior year and was named to the All-Southern team. I was invited to play in the State All-Star Game in Jackson, Mississippi, in the summer after graduating, but we had already moved to Gadsden, Alabama, and I had a summer job, so that was no longer an option.

Growing up, my Uncle Marshall told me endless stories about a football player by the name of "Goat" Hale doing marvelous things on the football field. One day during my senior year, I got a message from the school office that I had a visitor downstairs. I went down, and this athletic, gray-haired man stuck out his hand and said, "Hi, son, I am Goat Hale." I was awestruck, and I must have looked like a mental deficient. He told me that they had been watching me from over at Ole Miss, and he wanted to come back another day to talk about a scholarship. I don't think my feet touched the ground the remainder of the day.

My musical experiences followed along the same lines. I guess I started taking piano lessons when I must have been in the second or third grade. I learned from Mrs. Grady during school hours, since she was the grammar school music director and, of course, a friend of Mama's. We had a piano at home, where I practiced and learned my music. We had our recitals in the school auditorium, and they were dutifully attended by the parents and probably no one else. When I got to the seventh grade, I decided that I wanted to play an instrument and be in the band. Following in my father's footsteps, I guess. I wanted to learn to play the saxophone, but we had a trombone in the family, and l learned to play it. I am sorry that I gave up my piano lessons, but playing the trombone was going to lead me into a lot of fun.

Growing up next door to my paternal grandparents was a delightful experience. My grandmother spoiled me, and my grandfather was my best friend. It remained so until, crippled by small strokes, he succumbed to senility in his later years. One of the saddest moments in my life was when I visited him in his last year of life. He was confined to a bed in a nursing home, where it had been necessary to put him for the sake of Mama and Aunt Trudy, who had been looking after him for years. I went in to see him on a visit to Mobile, and he had no idea who I was. We had always been so close and had spent so much time together that it was hard to accept the loss of his warm love before the eventual loss from death.

When he died, we carried him back to Amory. Unbelievably, the funeral home in Amory is named Pickle Funeral Home for its founder, E. E. Pickle. It was operated by his son, Guy Pickle. The ghoulish humor never occurred to me until later in life. He lay in the parlor awaiting the funeral service, and when we turned to go into the chapel there suddenly came a loud, screaming cry, as if a feral animal were in extreme agony. My grandmother, who never raised her voice except in pique over some of Pa-pa's antics, wailed, "Goodbye, Dad." It was a poignant and somber moment indeed.

Pa-pa and I had many happy moments together when I was growing up. After starting school, just about every Friday night I was allowed to spend the night at my grandparents. That meant that I was going to be able to sleep with Pa-pa, and he would tell me stories about his being a cowboy and about his horse, "Old Cap." The stories never changed, but snakes grew longer, and the bulls got bigger and meaner every time the stories were told. Occasionally, he would tell Uncle Remus stories about Br'er Fox and Br'er Rabbit. I loved those tales, and I have been known to repeat them to my grandchildren.

Pa-pa and I fished together with cane poles and live bait until his infirmities made it impossible. Wherever we lived until I was in college, we fished whenever the opportunity presented itself. He was an excellent fisherman, and we rarely came home "skunked." On some occasions when we didn't catch anything, he would buy some fish off a fisherman who was having better luck. He referred to this as "using silver bait."

Usually on Saturdays after spending the night, I would get to go work with him. Most of the houses in those days were raised off the ground, and the plumbing lines were buried underneath the house, requiring the exposed pipes to be insulated against freezing. Usually, there was one person under the house taking measurements and another outside cutting the pipe to the proper length. My job was to crawl under the house with the piece of pipe and return with a new measurement. For this, I was paid the princely sum of a quarter a day. Later on, as I grew older and my knowledge grew as well, I was able to do the tasks of one of the other workers. One day Pa-pa and I were involved in putting pipe in a wall that was later going to be covered. Pa-pa was being careful to see that everything was straight, plumb, and just right. I exclaimed, "Pa-pa, why are we being so careful? No one is ever going to know if it is just right."

He replied, "I will." I never forgot that lesson.

Since my other grandparents lived about twenty miles away, I didn't get to see them as often. We would drive over every Sunday and spend the day with them. The Methodist church was one block up the street toward town. My grandmother usually sang in the choir, which was located in an empty space behind the pulpit. They didn't perform anthems but sang lustily through the hymns. Grandfather sat on the second row on the left. He always sat sideways while leaning back on the end of the pew, with his right arm draped over the back of the pew. He would sit there with his head tilted downward, and it was difficult to tell whether he had nodded off or not. However, when the preacher made a point that he particularly liked, his head would come up and in a resonant voice, he would intone, "Amen."

Supper was always served at six o'clock and consisted of leftovers from a large Sunday dinner. However, no one was allowed to sit down at the table until everyone was present. If someone were late, everyone waited until all else had arrived before they were seated. At the end of the meal my grandmother always asked, "Would you like something else, Presley?" He would always answer, "No, I've et sufficient."

After dinner everyone would retire to the front porch in complete darkness, except for the glow from my grandfather's pipe, fully loaded with George Washington crimp-cut tobacco. There were times when no one spoke, but we just sat there contemplating the serenity. After about an hour, we would get in our Model A Ford sedan and head home. I would try to stay awake, but I always succumbed to the lure of lying down on the back seat. When I fell asleep, I would be wakened from a bump or swerve and hope that we weren't too close to home as I was sleeping so well.

In the summertime I would spend a week at a time visiting, and to get there I was allowed to do something that no parent would permit nowadays. In order for me to have my bike up there, Mama would let me ride my bicycle the twenty miles to Shannon all alone. I would start out ahead of her, and I would take full advantage of the sights. I would stop on bridges over small streams and throw rocks at snakes in the shallow water below. The road across the bottom land, where the Tombigbee River flooded every spring, was flat and easy going. The roadbed was elevated about eight feet above the surrounding acreage and was always dry even in rainy season.

After a few miles the flat land ended, and low-level hills were the terrain of this area of the trip. This took up about fourteen miles of the road, until I would come to the small town of Nettleton. This was the home town of Aunt Trudie, Uncle Marshall's wife. It was also where Uncle Jim, Grandma Boozer's brother, owned a mercantile store. His son, Harrison, would graduate from Emery University with a degree in medicine later. On leaving Nettleton, the flat bottom land would start again, with the familiar raised roadbed insuring no flooded highway. A few miles outside Nettleton was an abandoned small silo, made of red clay tile and bricks. It had no top and was a small edifice when compared with silos in Iowa. One time a dead man was found inside, and some wag in Amory said he ran himself to death trying to find a corner to pee in. It was the town joke for years. A short distance down the road ended the trip, with Mama sitting on the front porch apparently worry-free.

In the mid-1930s, a horrendous tornado essentially wiped Tupelo, Mississippi, off the map. It hit early on a Sunday evening, just as we were preparing to go home from Shannon. It was dark and windy as we started out, but I don't remember much rain. Pap suddenly said, "Look up there; it looks like lights up in the sky," as he pointed toward Tupelo, nine miles to the north. We later learned that these were car lights being sucked up into the air by this killer storm. It was a devastating tornado, with enormous property damage and human lives lost. It did things like blow a small church, sitting on top of a hill, into a small pond at the bottom of the hill. This resulted in the death of the entire congregation in attendance that night. Later, as we drove through the devastation so often seen in the wake of tornadoes, we would see a city block completely without any buildings, save an old two-story red brick house probably constructed in the pre-civil war era.

This storm so frightened Miss Emma Lamb, who lived two doors up from my grandparents, that she began to live in a storm house she had built behind her home. This was simply a small cave dug into the side of a hill, which sloped down to the lower land on the rear of her property. The roof was simply dirt, about six feet thick, that remained from the excavation of the approximately eight-by-eight foot hole. The walls were also nothing but dirt, and the front was partly repacked dirt around a narrow wooden door. It was not a place that a person would build for a permanent residence, but was merely to dart into as a safe haven during stormy weather.

This was what Miss Emma would do for a while after the tornado, but eventually she became too afraid of a possible storm to venture out, even on a balmy day with clear, blue skies. Since the storm house had no facilities such as toilets, running water, facilities for cooking, bathing, or electricity, it was necessary for another person to come in to cook her meals, bring them to her, and take out the human waste in a slop jar. I don't know this from personal experience, but I understand she was not the most pleasant of souls inhabiting the earth. To solve her problem, she arranged that the Riley family would be bequeathed her house and land in Shannon along with her farm land on the outskirts of town in return for providing these services until her death.

The Rileys had a daughter who was the same age as my first cousin, Beth, Uncle Riley's daughter. They also had a son my age, Edward. We were fast buddies, so I was able to see a lot of this firsthand. In addition, Beth would occasionally help Lorraine, the daughter, to carry the meals to Miss Emma. A typical lunch would include an entire chicken, two large bowls of vegetables, a skillet of cornbread, and a dessert of some sort or another. This continued unabated for years.

As would be expected, with that amount of food consumed daily and no exercise, her weight and girth increased enormously. With no sun exposure and lack of hygiene, her skin began to break down with ulcers, abrasions, etc. Her health began to fail, and she died of complications these ailments. I am also certain that she must have had a severe vitamin D deficiency. When she died, they discovered a greater problem. She had gained so much weight they could not get her out of the storm house through the door. After consulting the powers that be, they just covered her up in the storm cellar, and she was thus buried on her own property. That was not an uncommon occurrence in those days.

Miss Emma's brother, Charlie, lived between my grandparents and Miss Emma. I don't really remember ever seeing his wife. I guess that she existed, but you couldn't prove it by me. I remember seeing Mr. Charlie walking out in his yard or walking by on his way to town. He was a short, little man who shuffled along with the aid of a cane. He had lower eyelids that rolled outward, which caused him to appear teary and extremely red-eyed. He had very white eyebrows which were never trimmed and a droopy white handlebar mustache that seemed to draw his face downward in a perpetual doleful expression. I don't recall ever hearing him say a single word. My grandmother called him "an old fool." Now, you must understand that my grandmother categorized men into either of three possibilities: they were four-square gentlemen, old fools, or white trash. She was quick to explain that there was nothing lower than white trash.

She was just as adamant about education. In her mind, there was just no excuse for not getting educated as much as your mind would carry you. I remember when Beth went off to college at Mississippi School for Women (MSCW), which was my grandmother's alma mater, and after about two weeks she called home and told Uncle Riley that she was coming home because she just hated it. Uncle Riley told her that was all right, but she would just have to go to another school. Of course she stayed, and there is now a Mary Elizabeth Boozer Brevard endowed chair at that school.

I can remember standing in my grandparent's front yard near the sidewalk and hearing the news from everyone that Japan had bombed Pearl Harbor. It was just at dusk, and it was getting difficult to see because of the impending darkness. It was an afternoon where my idyllic existence was taken away and my life was changed forever.

Things changed rapidly after that. Eligible young men were being drafted into the armed services, and increasingly, small banners were put into front windows with a blue star for each child that particular family had in the service. The radios were now playing music related to the war. They all were devoted to subjects like patriotism, separation of sweethearts with vows of being there when their lover returned, or how different life in the military was from back home. For some inductees from our area it was their first exposure to a balanced, nutritious diet, and it was immediately noticeable in sudden growth and muscular stature. For some it was their first time to have shoes that fit and were not worn-out hand-me-downs. Some individuals had built up calluses from years of ill-fitting shoes, but when they went into the service, the calluses were removed—and suddenly the limp they had for years was gone. At school, even we seventh graders were taught things that would be useful to us when we were put in the military. We learned to march, with all the various commands as column left, eyes right, etc. In some manner the school obtained some old World War I Springfield rifles. There weren't very many, but each male student was taught how to march with a rifle, the proper way to carry it, and basic skills such as present arms, etc. We were taught and performed exercises that were used by the army such, as jumping jacks and pushups. Without realizing, these forty-five minute marching, drilling, and in-place exercises had all the male seventh-grade students in good physical shape. Even the roly-poly boys began to demonstrate a waistline.

The next year, my dad bought a farm in the Tombigbee bottom land. A couple of years previously, both Jack and Rob had gone to Fort McClellan, Alabama, to get defense jobs as plumbers for considerably more money. They would eventually be sent to Huntsville, Alabama, to help build the Redstone Arsenal, where they were at this time. This would become, in later years, the NASA Space Program, where the Saturn Rocket that propelled the first lunar program and landing was made.

At that time, it was building barracks, mess halls, and latrines that required numbers of plumbers far beyond the capability that the local plumbing union could provide. Jack's and Rob's employment provided the astronomical wage of $1.50 an hour. No one had ever heard of such money for doing plumbing. But at this time Pap went into the farming business with the same enthusiastic zeal that he usually showed for new projects. The fact was the only thing he knew about farming was that he lived next door to and was good friends with Joel Rogers, who was a farmer.

I have noticed that a lot of men in their mid-lives wanted to live the life of a farmer. This was substituted for having a mid-life crisis. He did have a sharecropper on the place who often made very strong suggestions about what to do with the farm. Pap bought a W-2 Allis Chalmers tractor with all the attachments, such as plows, discs, cultivators, harvesters, etc. I was twelve years old at the time and finishing up my seventh-grade year. I vividly recall going down to the tractor place with my dad and picking up our new tractor. I had been driving our Ford pickup around the yard, but I was far from being skilled at it. Nevertheless, my dad put me up on the tractor and away I went, driving it down the highway, over the Tombigbee River Bridge, to its new home in our brand new tractor shed.

I became very proficient at handling that old tractor through that summer. I spent my pre-eighth-grade summer working as a farmhand who knew about as much about farming as Pap did. I learned to plow and disc fields, plant crops, hoe cotton, clear new ground before the days of power saws, walk behind a mule pulling a plow, and run the harvester over oats, vetch, and some summer wheat. Thankfully, we had very good year farming. We made over a bale of cotton to the acre, filled the cribs with corn, and did well all the way around. The problem was that the initial outlay was far more than the input.

The sad fact was that the money that Jack and Rob were making began to look very enticing. Eventually we lost the farm and Pap had to sell our house, the cabinet business, and all other assets that could be sold to raise money to clear the debt. Right before the Christmas holidays, we packed up the belongings that we had left and headed for the unknown in Huntsville, Alabama.

Through all of this, my mother never let us children see her crying, though I am sure that she probably did a lot of it. It must have been heartrending for her to leave the pleasant life she and Pap had built there, and to leave the home she had made in the house that her father had built for her. She kept her outward appearance of tranquility and her easy laugh. Many years later, the mother and daughter who lived next door to my parents dropped by to see me in my workshop. The conversation turned to Mama, and they talked about getting up early in the morning and hearing my mother's laugh coming from her open windows next door. The mother said that her daughter asked, "What is she laughing at?"

She replied, "Life."

Thus, we departed Amory and all of its comforts, and the nomadic part of my life began.

Chapter 4

World War II and College — My World Changes

Huntsville was not prepared for the sudden inflow of workers who suddenly appeared to build the arsenal and did not have all the ancillary facilities that were needed to accommodate the hordes of workers. Because Rob had gotten to the town earlier, before the scarcity of housing was clearly manifest, he was able to get settled in a nice second-floor apartment in the downtown area. Late that summer Jack's draft number had come up and he had been inducted into the armed forces, getting his choice of service in the Army Air Corps. By the time we arrived in Huntsville, housing was a thing you wanted but was nowhere to be found.

By this time, Marshall had resigned his teaching and coaching job in Hamilton, Alabama. and had headed to Huntsville. Pa-pa had closed his business and had a supervisor's position waiting for him. Now we were on the road headed to the same place. The trip up made us look like some of the Okies described by Steinbeck in *The Grapes of Wrath*. There was our old 1940 Ford pickup, loaded to the gills, but which no longer belonged to us. Benton Lantrip, the fellow who worked in Pap's cabinet shop, bought it and drove it to Huntsville loaded with our furniture, helped unload it, and refused to accept any payment except gas money. Gas then was twenty-five cents a gallon for regular. He followed us in our 1940 Mercury sedan that did still belong to us.

The trip from Amory to Huntsville is not all that long, but the speed limit all over the country was thirty-five miles per hour in an effort to increase the mileage made on a gallon of gas. In addition there was gas rationing, with weekly limits available based on your priority. If you were a normal citizen, you were given an A sticker to put on your windshield, which entitled you to three gallons of gasoline a week. If you drove a pickup truck, you got a T sticker, which allowed you five gallons a week. If you drove a car or truck that was involved in the war effort, you would receive a different sticker that enabled you to increased gasoline, dependent on the need for your position.

In order to make a trip, a traveler had to essentially park his or her car or truck and save up gas coupons until he or she had sufficient gallons to make the trip. It effectively cut out joy rides. At any rate, we eventually arrived in Huntsville and were able to see where we would be living. Before we arrived, Marshall, Pa-pa and Pap had purchased a small house in the Mayfair subdivision. These were small, quickly constructed, but well-built houses solely made to take care of the influx of people arriving daily. They only used three different house plans, I'm sure for the sake of expediency; but it resulted in a homeowner being able to pick out a clone of the family house up and down the street without difficulty. Ma-ma said it reminded her of a pauper's graveyard, where all the tombstones were alike. Nowadays these are known as tract housing.

The plan for our housing was for all three families to live in this single house. The costs and house payments would be split three ways, and the ration cards would be pooled and used as needed for the whole. We had one bedroom, while Marshall, Trudie, and their daughter, Barbara Ann, had the other bedroom; Ma-ma and Pa-pa had the living room. The meals were prepared by the women in some sort of agreed arrangement, and everyone got fed daily without any noticeable friction. There was no TV in those days. The entertainment was the radio, and in your space in the house you could listen to what you wanted, as long as it was not loud. It was truly a communal effort. Karl Marx would have been proud of us. However, there was one fly in this communistic enterprise—there was only one bathroom.

For a teenage boy with the desire for personal privacy exploding in his own little world, this arrangement presented problems. To move from a home of our own to all of the family being in one small, ten-by-ten foot room took a lot of getting acclimated. The first thing we learned was just to accept the situation. No one was taking more than their share of space, and there was nothing to gain by moping and griping. If we brooded on the lack of space and privacy or complained about the living accommodations, it served no purpose except to put everyone on edge. There seemed to be a tacit understanding that no one would stay in the house unless there were chores to be done. Everyone else stayed out of the house and did things where there was space—outside. The men left for work very early in the morning and did not return until very late in the afternoon. The first one home got his or her bath, dressed, and moved outside or returned to his or her assigned space. The women cooked, fed the families, and saw that the children were bathed, gotten ready for bed, and into assigned rooms early in the evening. I went to school early in the morning on a municipal bus. I ate lunch at the school cafeteria, and after school went to the YMCA with my buddies. There we played games, tennis, etc. until time to catch the bus home for supper, bath, and school homework. Everyone went to his or her own area at night and avoided making noise. Weekends were spent doing things together away from home. Pa-pa and I did a lot of fishing, which I thought was great. It was a pattern of life that no one enjoyed but everyone tolerated without fussing. One thing we did know, it was not going to be like this forever.

The atmosphere of the world was completely changed by this time in the war. The entire focus of America was the winning of the two-front war, and this was quickly woven into the everyday fabric of our lives. The military was ever-present in Huntsville, and its citizens were constantly running upon military convoys. If a person came upon a convoy on the road, she was stuck behind them until they or the delayed party turned off. Convoys only went thirty miles per hour instead of the normal speed limit of thirty-five, and this discrepancy could be maddening to a teenager like me when following a convoy. If unlucky enough to come upon one from a side road, then the traveler was really out of luck. It was a case of patiently, or impatiently, sitting there and waiting for the convoy to make its snail-like progression until clearing the road.

As hard as it is to believe, there were people in the United States who were Nazi sympathizers and constantly worked against the war movement. The populace was constantly being warned against innocently giving out small bits of information that could be paired with other innocent small bits of information to give up a vital piece of information to the enemy. Posters were everywhere warning, "Loose lips lose ships."

Of course, the paranoia of being spied upon led to some comical conclusions. In Birmingham, Alabama, a man had a home on the crest of Red Mountain and installed a flagpole in his front yard, probably as a patriotic gesture. Every day, he would run the American flag up the flagpole, and dutifully, every night he carefully took the flag down. Many people in Birmingham were convinced he was a German spy, and that he was sending signals with his flag raising and lowering every day. I guess it never occurred to them that there were much more sophisticated ways of sending spy information than raising or lowering a flag.

As the result of the war effort, the economy of the United States was vastly improving. It took World War II to really end the Great Depression. This was not the result of the twenty-one dollars a month that a buck private earned in the Army, but because of the need to furnish him with the things to fight with and to transport them to him.

Mobile, Alabama, was a beehive of activity, constructing freighters for ocean transport. There, ships were being welded together instead of riveted, and pipes were being welded together instead of being threaded and fastened together with large metal flanges, gaskets, and bolts. Ships were turned out at an amazing rate of speed and met the needs for transportation of war goods. Not only did they construct enough ships to make up for the loss of merchant steamers due to German U-Boats, but they surpassed that, which allowed increased materials to be landed overseas. The factories were "manned" by females and older males. All of this cost money, which was paid by the government with bond sales and with the increased tax money that came in as a result of increased spending by the populace. The funding of the war was a masterpiece, and is a subject unto itself. The manning of the factories with female workers was revolutionary for the times, and was the first step in the demise of stay-at-home moms. It was very much like the song about the dough boys in World War I, later featured by George M. Cohan, "How you gonna keep 'em down on the farm, after they've seen Paree?"

With all the conscription of young males and females into the armed services, there was an insidious happening that no one really noticed. All the young male physicians were being drafted or were voluntarily entering the war effort. The same was happening with nurses. Suddenly there were only older medical personnel to care for the civilian population, which greatly outnumbered the military, where all the young medical workers were going. The poor remaining physicians were grossly overworked. Looking at pictures of all the old physicians working then, one can see the fatigue permanently etched on their faces.

Up until this time, hospitals were essentially run by physicians solely for the care of patients. That was the sole function of any or all hospitals. There were very few public hospitals, but most were owned by physicians, churches, etc. The few county and state hospitals were operated for the care of the indigent. No matter who owned the hospital, physicians were in command of the day-to-day operation of that institution. The head physician was usually called the chief-of-staff and he was the head honcho. There was also the director of nursing, who ran all the services of the day-to-day operations with an iron fist of control that would make a drill sergeant quaver. In the Catholic hospitals, this function was served by the head nun, and most of the nurses were nuns.

Suddenly this all changed. Doctors and nurses were so scarce and busy that no one had the time and energy to see to the day-to-day routine of a well-run patient-care facility. Very innocently, business people were hired to fill this void, and the hospital administrator was born. Before anyone recognized the fact, the camel had its nose under the tent and was now fully occupying it. It has never been banished to the outside since then. Business established control of the management of hospitals as the result of a very innocently devised move to enable the continuation of civilian patient care despite a world war. This left the hospital administrator trying to serve two masters: financial interests and compassionate patient care. No man can serve two masters, and it is not yet recognized that this is an impossible task.

Into all of this organized chaos of wartime upheaval, families were held together and children were educated as always. Thus I began my second semester of the ninth grade at Huntsville High School, not really truly aware of all of these other things going on around me. Huntsville High was a much larger school than Amory High. The students were very open and friendly, and I quickly made friends to pal around with before and after school. One of my buddies was on the debate team. It had never occurred to me that boys would participate in something like that. At Amory, only girls participated in things like debate teams and glee clubs. It was difficult for me to consider being part of such a thing. Boys were in the band or on athletic teams, but never in sissy things.

I was pleased to find that I was as advanced in class work as the students in the new school. I had been prepared very well. I joined the band, and they were glad to get another trombone player. We also spent one hour every day making airplane models that were given to people who found it necessary to identify airplanes by sight, such as airplane spotters, air cadets training to be pilots, etc. We made both solid models cut from balsa wood and models made with balsa wood skeletons that were covered with tissue paper sheets attached by airplane glue. After attaching, the paper was wet and allowed to dry. If the builder did a reasonably good job of getting it on smoothly, the paper would shrink and become taut and wrinkle free. All of the models were painted black, so that both enemy and friendly airships could be identified by the silhouette alone. I really did enjoy that class.

That spring, there was a prom held in the school gym. I didn't know what a prom was and had to ask Mama. Of course I went stag, along with some of my buddies from the ninth grade. Suddenly I realized that there was a real band playing the dance music. This was not some little high school band; this was the Auburn Knights. I was totally mesmerized by the experience. I don't know if they were really as good as I remember, but they had an excellent reputation. During the dance, the lead trombone stood and played a solo. That was the best thing I had ever heard. I stayed 'til the end of the dance and never left the bandstand. I remember thinking, "Boy, wouldn't it be great to play in a band like that!" Little did I know that was to be part of my destiny.

The following summer, I got my first job as a first-year plumber's apprentice. The business agent for Local 495 of the plumbers and steamfitters union, Mr. Bob Hadaway, gave the okay for me to work as a first-year apprentice. This was mainly on the pull of my Dad, Pa-pa, and uncles, who were held in high esteem by the people in the trade for their quality of work and their work ethic. Marshall, Dad, and I worked on a housing project that was being built for low-income renters. My job entailed what I had been doing for Pa-pa for years. A first-year apprentice in those days made fifty cents an hour, and it went further than the seven-plus dollars that is the minimum for an hourly wage today. Thus is the wisdom of politicians.

Every summer since then, from my first year, I worked in the plumbing field until my third year of medical school. Each year I made a little more than the previous year, as I advanced through second, third, etc. years, until I "turned out" as plumber after my fifth year of apprenticeship. This was after my first year of medical school and to say the least, I was accustomed to taking exams. There was some rumbling and grumbling from other apprentices, as I had only spent five summers, not five full years, doing apprentice work.

Pap told me that some of them were actively looking forward to my falling on my face when I took my journeyman's exam. Pap gave me four small books about plumbing, written by Starbuck, which could be used for studying for the exam. I skimmed over them, but I had been doing this since I was five years old and didn't see too much in the books that I wasn't acquainted with. The exam was given at night, so I didn't hear how I did until the next day. Pap called me the next day from work and told me I had made 100 percent on the exam. It was the first and last time that anyone made that score. Of course, it was the first and last time that they had someone who had just finished two semesters preparing for exams in medical school take the test.

The next year, we moved back to Mississippi while Pap went on a job in Texas. Actually, I went to Amory because Mama wasn't exactly enamored with the school system in Shannon, where she and Tom went to spend the year with her folks. In the meantime, Mama and Pa-pa had moved back to Amory, where Pa-pa had another supervisor's job on the construction of a defense facility in Prairie, Mississippi, which was only a short drive from their home.

Pap came back the next year and we moved to Gadsden, Alabama, where Pap worked on an addition to the Goodyear Rubber Co. tire plant. I also worked there in my usual summer plumbing job. Housing was scarce in Gadsden also, but Pap found and rented one side of a small duplex in East Gadsden. Again, we were cramped, but not as cramped as before. Now we had a real living room and two bedrooms, so only Tom and I shared a room. A kitchen with a small dinette area rounded out the living space. At least the one bathroom wasn't occupied all the time. In addition, every unit had a sturdy clothesline outside, as washing machines and driers weren't available in our world. I went to Gadsden High School my junior year. I played fullback on the football team, but unfortunately, I experienced a high ankle sprain before the season opened. It took a long time to heal well, and I got very little playing time until the latter part of the season. I played enough to earn my football letter, but it was nothing to write home about.

I went back to Amory for my senior year and lived with Ma-ma and Pa-pa again because Pap thought he was going to have to go to another job out of town. It turned out he didn't, but I stayed at Amory my senior year in high school. I returned to Gadsden that summer and again spent the summer on another addition to the Goodyear plant. By now Pap had bought a small house in East Gadsden that was very similar to the one we had in Huntsville. The difference was there was only one family in the house, and now there was a small dining room.

One day on the job Pap and I were eating our lunch, and Pap turned to me and said, "I want you to watch the brick masons on this job because we are going to build a concrete block garage in our backyard." I had watched them in a superficial way prior to this but had never watched them closely. Shortly thereafter, we went down to a building supply house and purchased enough concrete blocks to build a two-car garage. This was going to be Pap's second garage to hold tools but never a car. After it was built and we moved tools into it, it was called a shop; but prior to that time, we were always building a garage.

We laid out the floor area on the ground and installed the forms to hold the concrete. Pap arranged for the delivery of the concrete on an afternoon when he would be at work. He was depending on Tom and me to screed it and rough trowel it for the final finish. Well, the concrete came, but Tom was nowhere to be found. I discovered that he had wheedled Mama into letting him go play baseball with his buddies. There I was, with a cement truck full of concrete and no help. It builds character, they say. The truck driver felt sorry for me, and against company rules helped me do the rough screed work so at least it was all pretty much the same thickness. Although it could never be said that the floor was smooth, no one ever tripped over an unexpected rise or fall in the floor.

I would like to say it was good planning, but really it was only good fortune that I started to lay my first blocks on the back corner. It took me about two courses before I figured out the method for being sure that the block was perfectly perpendicular, as well as level, before setting it on the wet mortar. By the time that I reached the front, I had gotten pretty good at it. Before we got all the way around, Pap had added an additional small space on the side to hold paints, lacquers, etc. I hadn't built that side before then, so it just meant leaving a place in the wall for a door. The small addition also had a concrete floor, but I had help this time, so the final product was much more like a concrete floor ought to be. The final product had a single door on the back (later a storage shed for stacking and drying of lumber was added), two windows on one side, and double doors on the front. Pap began buying new tools (may of which are still in use today), and soon a real woodworking shop appeared.

I had waited to get home to Gadsden before applying to the University of Alabama for admission to the freshman class of 1946. They had assured us not to worry; there would be adequate space for everyone. The day finally came when we packed my belongings and headed to the university in Tuscaloosa. As expected, the place was overrun with returning war veterans, and again I was faced with a housing shortage. The regular dorms were all full, including the crumbling old dorm where Pap had once lived. They were using the barracks in an old abandoned military station for the overflow housing needs. I fell into this category.

By the time I had gotten out there and entered, I could see that their remodeling effort barely went past sweeping the place out and moving in cots. The rooms were long with cots aligned perpendicular to the outer wall, just like the ones in the Army. There was no privacy available and no quiet study area available, either. I took one look and told my parents, "I'm not going to stay here." I knew that I was (and still am) very shy in crowds, and I could not learn in a situation with no privacy available. We packed up and went back to Gadsden.

The next day, Mama called Aunt Trudy and discussed the matter with her. She remembered that Jacksonville State Teachers College was just twenty-two miles away, and they were expanding their curriculum to meet the needs of incoming veterans. The following day, we were on the road to Jacksonville, and I enrolled and was able to schedule every class that I needed without difficulty. To solve the housing problem, they were helpful in finding me a ride with some other commuters from Gadsden. I rode over every morning and came back that afternoon with a bunch of absolutely fine people.

I liked staying at home. It gave me a place to study, and I enjoyed living with my entire family again. It also gave me time in the afternoons and on weekends to work on the job of constructing the garage–shop. Besides that, I didn't miss anything on the campus, as there was little going on since most of the veterans were married with families where they spent their idle moments. At first, it was odd to see so many fellows roaming the campus with various prostheses, false eyes and obvious war wounds. Soon such sights became mundane.

I was well into my freshman year when we received a call from someone in Shannon, calling to tell us that my grandfather had walked home from work, gone into the second bedroom, began warming himself by the glowing Warm Morning heater, collapsed, and died without saying a word. We loaded up the car and I drove to Shannon. On the way, Mama called from the backseat in a very soft voice, "Are you sure that they said it was Daddy who died?" She was extremely close to her dad. That night I slept well, and we buried my grandfather the next day.

We drove back to Gadsden, but soon began to hear that my maternal grandmother had Alzheimer's disease. In those days, it was called senile dementia. It was patently obvious that Uncle Riley couldn't take care of her by himself, so she moved in with us. At that time she wasn't in too much confusion, but would have spells when she wouldn't know who we were. This gradually worsened with time. She had an insatiable desire to walk. She had no particular place that she wanted to go, but she just wanted to be on the move. She slept on a cot in the living room, and we always made sure that the doors were securely fastened so she could not wander off.

She liked to ride, and on recreational jaunts she would see a billboard and ask us, "Who is this old fool, Dr. Pepper, who is always advertising?" After a while she just became more than the family could manage, and she was hospitalized. She died in a few short months. People could not understand what could have possibly caused her mental deterioration. It was the prevailing view amongst the theorists of the family that it could be traced to the thick black coffee, which always sat on the back of her kitchen wood stove, that she drank all day, every day. It was as good a theory as any, I guess.

The remainder of my freshman year went by uneventfully. I knew that I had to make good grades, and I did. My sophomore year saw increased extracurricular activities beginning to occur on campus. The music department began to increase greatly with new faculty, programs, and student enrollment. They started a marching and concert band, and I decided to join. I began to become more involved with the music programs, and it became obvious that I needed to move full time onto the campus. I moved into Farney Hall on the old campus. It required a walk of about a mile to get to the main campus, but walking didn't bother me in those days.

An added bonus was that the dorm supervisor was "Doc" Gary, who would wind up teaching me essentially all of my chemistry classes. He would also hire me for the position of laboratory assistant, which provided me with pocket change I wouldn't have had otherwise. He was a very kind, gentle, and learned man who had the knack of making complicated science easy. He reminded me very much of Mr. Chips in the play *Goodbye, Mr. Chips*. He was from Midway, Alabama, where his family was made up of rather wealthy farmers. There was his childhood home, and it was apparently a classical southern mansion. He had fond memories of the place and would talk about it often. He kept a lot of his family heirlooms in his single room in Farney Hall. Often the school would ask for the loan of some of these, such as silver punch bowls, silver candelabra, etc.

I soon became very interested in the extracurricular activity of joining a dance band. In those days, the music was the big band sound. An orchestra usually consisted of five saxophones, three trumpets, three trombones, and a four-man rhythm section. The saxophone section ordinarily consisted of two altos, two tenors, and a baritone sax. This varied from band to band, depending on the sound desired. All of this section usually doubled on clarinet and, sometimes, flute. The brass section consisted of first, second, and third trumpets and trombones. The first trumpets and trombones ordinarily carried the melody and second and third chairs provided the harmony, with the second chairs usually playing all the solos. Rhythm sections consisted of piano, string bass (bull fiddle), drums, and guitar. This section was indispensable, as it set the tempo for every piece played. Being in a dance band was something that had intrigued me since my experience with the Auburn Knights in the ninth grade.

In my sophomore year there was an influx of musical students from the surrounding areas, mostly Anniston and Gadsden. One fellow who matriculated into the school at this time, Johnny Long, was a very different sort of guy with the determination to be a superior musician and conductor. He was from the town of Guntersville,

Alabama, and had been a musician and conductor even before he graduated from high school. The band director at Guntersville High had been drafted when Johnny was in the eleventh grade. There was no one to take his place, so Johnny did. He held the band together and was the band director, unofficially of course, for two years.

I don't know what happened to the program after he graduated. He was a student at Jacksonville State, and at the same time, he was band director of the Jacksonville High school band. He decided that he wanted to start a dance band of his own, and that is what he did. He started putting players together from the college and high school. I really don't remember how I got into the band. I just remember being in the band at rehearsals very soon after he formed the orchestra.

Johnny was a taskmaster and a stickler for playing music exactly correct. This quickly turned us into a pretty good unit, and we began to get dates to play. People drifted in and out of the band as events dictated. We had some professional musicians at different time periods. One of these musicians was an older fellow who played lead alto sax for us. Before starting to play with us, he had been a member of the Ted Weems' Band, a professional band that was very popular at the time. I may have discovered what caused his transfer. I noticed that before we began playing at every dance, he would stash a fifth of whiskey behind his music stand. At the end of the dance the bottle would be empty, but I never, ever saw him take a sip. It never seemed to affect his playing, either.

Johnny went on to be the band director of many high schools and ultimately, he received his doctorate and became head of the music department at Troy University. He remained the band director, and the last I saw him, he and his band were the halftime show at the Senior Bowl. I went down on the field and spoke to him. I haven't seen or heard from him since then, though I have thought of him often.

During all of this, I also was asked to join the school symphony orchestra as first trombonist. The orchestra was under the direction of Fritz Heim, who had been concert master for the Sigmund Romberg orchestra. He was a flamboyant man and a remarkable musician and violinist. It was from this experience of playing the classics that I became an avid fan of classical music. I was playing first trombone in the marching and concert bands, the symphony orchestra, and Johnny's band. I was having a delightful time and was enjoying every moment that I played music. I began to consider switching my major to music, but after a Dutch uncle talk with myself, I had to admit that I just didn't have the talent for that career. I surely did have an awful lot of fun playing for dances all over the South almost every weekend, and an awful lot of Wednesdays. For some reason, clubs with only adults held dances on Wednesday nights.

All through school I continued to work each summer as a plumber, and I usually could get temporary work during extended holidays like Christmas, Thanksgiving, and spring break. My dance band job was also a large contributor to the college fund. I ordinarily made fifteen dollars a dance. Now, before you turn up your nose at that meager sum of money, let me remind you that in today's dollar value that would amount to around a hundred-and-fifty dollars. At any rate, all of this accumulated, so that I was able to pay for the vast majority of my college costs without having to rely too much on my parents.

This was important because my brother, Tom, was about to start at Georgia Tech, which would require paying extra as an out-of-state student. We made it without anyone having to borrow money, not even a dime. I am pretty sure that was true for Tom also. I continued doing this plumbing work until I was a junior in medical school. My last plumbing job was in Childersburg, Alabama, where they added an extension on a rayon plant. The next summer, I was able to work in the medical field, and I was through with plumbing as a trade, for which I am eternally grateful. I was not interested in being a plumber all of my remaining life. There was nothing wrong with being a plumber; heaven knows that all of my family were plumbers. I just didn't like it well enough to spend the rest of my life doing it.

I continued to do well with my studies, and I began to close in on taking all my required studies. I had to take physics my junior year, which required having a lab partner. I got paired up with this cute little black-headed girl named Nancy Harper. My grandchildren know her better as Nanny. We suffered through physics lab, such as drying off ice in a room with no air-conditioning, in order to measure the number of calories of heat given off when ice melts. Getting the ice to melt was absolutely no problem, but getting it dry before it started to melt was quite a problem. We started dating, and soon it became a steady thing. We would marry in August, 1950, before I started medical school in September.

I applied for medical school at Alabama and nowhere else. For some reason, I never considered not getting in. I did discuss this with my dad and sort of made provisional plans to go to graduate school at Emery if I didn't get in. I went down to Birmingham for my interview with the admissions committee, and it went very smoothly. I had a car this time, as Nancy's dad let me use his to drive down. Nancy lived at home while going to school, as she was a "local." Therefore, I got to know her parents very well.

It was not long after that I got a letter from Alabama, telling me that I was accepted as a member of the 1950 freshman class. I remember being very excited and elated over being accepted, but it didn't impress me that much. I just felt as if it were something that was going to happen, and I shouldn't get all big-headed about it. It was a very peculiar feeling, and I thanked God for my good fortune. Later, when I found that I was one of fifty selected out of 2,500 applicants, I felt more grateful.

As usual, I worked at my summer plumbing job, this time on a high-rise bank building in Macon, Georgia. Pap was superintendent of the job, and both Tom and I had jobs. I was an apprentice plumber and Tom was an apprentice welder. We all lived together in one side of a rented duplex for the last time.

Nancy and I were married in the First Methodist Church of Jacksonville in August. Since it was too late to apply for a job in the Birmingham and Jefferson county school systems, she kept her job in Gadsden, and I went on to live in the medical school dorms at school. Another new life was beginning.

Chapter 5

Medical School — It Wasn't All Hard Work, Just Most of It

The medical school that existed when I attended my first class in Birmingham was not a new school of medicine. The University of Alabama had offered a two-year school for many years. People would enroll, and after finishing the two years they would transfer to other schools to finish their third and fourth years. Dr. Tinsley Harrison often said that the practice of medicine in Alabama was of higher quality than many other states because students were always transferred into, and graduated from, very good universities. At that time, it was amazing how many practicing physicians were graduates of Harvard, Johns Hopkins, etc.

The two-year school was located on the campus in Tuscaloosa when the war ended. Suddenly the facilities were flooded with requests from returning veterans for not only admittance to medical school, but for the school to become a four-year school. There was a march on the state capitol in Montgomery to demand a state school be provided that could award MD degrees. In order to obtain such a goal, there had to be clinical facilities to see and hospitalize patients, research laboratories for the faculty, and a source of patients that could be used for clinical teaching. This was far beyond the physical and manpower capabilities of the university campus at Tuscaloosa.

To solve this problem, the medical school was moved to Birmingham. Jefferson County had just finished a seventeen-story building next to the old Hillman Hospital to serve the indigent population; it was known as The Jefferson-Hillman Hospital Complex. The Hillman building supposedly was not allowed to house hospital patients, but it did contain the emergency room and labor and delivery facilities with pre- and postpartum wards on the fifth floor. The patient load for the Jefferson hospital was not heavy enough to require all the floors to be potential patient areas, and some floors were changed to classrooms, student labs, offices, and faculty laboratories.

All faculty members that had taught the courses in the first two years of medical school were moved from Tuscaloosa to Birmingham. Faculty members for the clinical years were recruited from all around America. Dr. Champ Lyons was recruited from Tulane to be head of surgery. Dr. Kendrick Hare, an Alabama native from Marion Junction, came from Cornell to be head of pediatrics. Dr. Nick Jones and Dr. James Garber were recruited from their private practices in Birmingham to be the heads of gynecology and obstetrics, respectively.

By far the largest prize was the recruitment of Dr. Tinsley Harrison to be the head of internal medicine. Dr. Harrison came to help with the formation of the four-year school because of the love he had for Alabama, as only a native son could have. Dr. Harrison originally became renowned because of his book, *Failure of the Circulation*, in the 1930s. This detailed the changes that occurred in the human body as the result of heart failure. These changes that he so clearly enunciated are only recently being appreciated by cardiologists because of the recent pharmaceutical developments of alpha and beta blockers. By the time that he came to Alabama, his textbook, *Harrison's Principles of Internal Medicine,* was used by essentially all the medical schools as their preferred textbook on internal medicine. His appointment brought immediate legitimacy to the Alabama school. When Dr. Crocker, the first four-year school dean, died suddenly from a coronary occlusion, Dr. Harrison served as interim dean. But he soon got back to doing what he loved—taking care of patients, teaching medical students and house staff, and continuing his many facets of cardiac research. As you can tell, he was one of my medical heroes.

I moved into the medical school dorms up the street from the hospital. Each area was assigned to medical fraternities, but the assignment of rooms was not on the basis of fraternity affiliation.

There was a big-screen TV set in the parlor, and this allowed me to become acquainted with television. It was the first time that I had ever been able to sit and watch it. All I had seen of it before were glimpses in store windows and in an occasional restaurant.

I roomed with a charming fellow, John T. Moore, who was a senior, an ardent lover of opera and foreign films, and the most dedicated soul I have ever known to his announced goal of practicing medicine in his small home town. He was a superb roommate and a great source of information about what lay ahead for me. He would drag me off to opera movies and foreign films. There was a theater on the south side that showed this sort of thing. He had a car, and I had enough money to afford a ticket. I learned to appreciate opera, and I became a fan of Alec Guinness when he was only being shown in foreign film theaters in black and white.

When we both got fed up with eating hospital food, we would use his car to drive downtown to Britling's Cafeteria. The money problem limited the choosing of food, but it surely did beat hospital food by a long way. During these times together, he explained to me how important it was to never fall behind in any class because they moved at such a fast clip that one could never catch back up. He also stressed that if I kept up with the classwork, on the night before an exam I should very briefly go over my notes to refresh my brain and then go to a movie. I did this all through medical school, and it worked like a charm. I would be fresh and bushy-tailed, and a lot of my classmates would come in bleary-eyed and obviously all jazzed up from drinking strong coffee all night. It wasn't hard to figure who was going to make the high scores.

So, this was the school that I entered in September, 1950. The first day was relatively insignificant. We reported first to biochemistry. We were told what was expected from us as a class and as an individual. We were taken to the biochemistry lab and assigned our lab space. We went next to micro anatomy, where the process more or less repeated itself. That afternoon we went to gross anatomy.

Now, every school has one course that is used to separate the sheep from the goats. At Alabama this course was gross anatomy. The class previous to us was acclaimed by the Dean to be the best class ever admitted to the school. Seven of the fifty students failed, with gross anatomy being the main culprit. You can be sure that everyone in our class was acutely aware of these facts. In fact, it became such a stressful force in our lives, Dr. Boyer of the anatomy department called the class together and told us that we as a whole had to relax a little bit. He explained that we could probably memorize all the facts in our textbook, but if we did, our brain would be so full of facts that we wouldn't be able to remember our phone numbers. Everyone relaxed and laughed, and anatomy became a lot easier after that.

We reported to the gross anatomy lab that afternoon. The lab was on the top floor of a wing of the hospital. It had no windows, except for small decorative fan lights located just under the ceiling. There were about fourteen stainless steel boxes on pipe legs, situated down either side of the walls. These boxes were located perpendicular to the long walls, but were placed so that there was ample room for four people to work, with two students on each side.

We all gathered in the front of the lab, and Dr. Boyer explained in plain terms the rules of behavior in the laboratory. There would be no loud and boisterous behavior allowed, the cadavers would always be treated with the utmost respect, and anyone found removing any body part from the lab would be summarily dismissed from school, permanently. Everyone seemed to understand all of that without difficulty. We were assigned our spaces, with four students to each cadaver. I worked with Gilbert Melson, who would die in a single engine plane crash not too long after graduating. On the other side were two fellows that were Sewanee University graduates, and apparently they had been former classmates.

The tank that held the cadaver was about seven-feet long and about three-feet wide. The depth of the tank was about two feet, and the top of the box was closed by two hinged doors that spanned the width and hung down along the sides when opened. They instructed us to open the tanks, and there was the body of a male, approximately fifty years of age, stocky in build but not obese, with his arms folded sedately across his abdomen. He was hoisted to tabletop height by pulling down levers at each end of the tank that locked in place to secure the raised platform. His head had been shaved prior to death, but there was a short stubble of hair that had grown back, postmortem. Closer observation revealed burn marks around the skull and encircling both wrists and ankles. It was obvious that he had been electrocuted as a cause of death. We were standing there, just looking down on him, when one of the Sewanee boys said, "You know, I've seen dead people before, but no one this dead."

We were all required to wear brown full-length lab coats whenever we were in the lab. We learned that day that whenever we left the sanctity of the lab wearing our light brown lab coats, we would be shunned by anyone in the vicinity. That day, we had to wet rags in some sort of tissue preservative that reeked with formaldehyde. We wrapped our cadaver with these wet rags to prevent him from drying out, but when we left the lab the horrible smell went with us. It soon became evident that our lab coats were permanently saturated with the odor. From then on, when we got on the freight elevator (which we were required to use) and rode the sexteen floors up or down, if anyone was on the elevator, they got off; if anyone stopped the car to get on, they let us pass. I remember things on the elevator that would occasionally bring levity into the situation, like the sign posted one day on the wall of the car proclaiming an impending dance that was going to have as a door prize, "A Genuine Simulated Diamond."

The laboratory was the province of Rufus. He was a medical student in the class ahead of us. If you needed to know anything or just needed anything, you asked Rufus. He dissected the "practical," which was a demonstration cadaver, located at the front of the room where Rufus would have done today's dissection yesterday. If anyone were having trouble with his dissection, he could go look and attempt to make his cadaver look the same way.

Another of Rufus's chores was to gather all the cadavers that were donated to the university and to make sure that they were properly handled and stored for the next class. The state penal and mental institutions were large providers of donated bodies. People who had been incarcerated for many years would die, and their family members would be in a quandary about what to do with the body of a family member who was barely known by the surviving relatives. The state would acquire these bodies, and after assuring the family that it would be treated with utmost respect and provided a Christian burial, they would accept the cadaver as a donation. I don't know if the families got a tax break or not.

Well, one day Rufus got a notice from the mental institution at Mount Vernon, Alabama, that it had five bodies to be picked up. The university owned an old panel truck that was used for such things. It was the same truck that we used to travel to patients' homes when we were on home delivery in our senior year. We drove it in case we had to transport the delivering mother to the hospital because of unexpected complications with the delivery. Rufus signed out the truck and drove down to Mount Vernon. This was before the days of interstates, so he was traveling on two-lane state highways through mostly rural areas. He picked up the five bodies and was driving back on Highway 5.

Just after passing through Pine Level, where Highway 10 crosses Highway 5, there is a stop sign that clearly signifies who has the right of way. Rufus was tooling through this intersection when a local citizen ran the stop sign and smashed into the side of the old panel truck just behind the rear wheel. This caused the truck to start spinning, and the centrifugal force caused the back door to fly open; bodies then began spewing forth from the rear of the truck. When everything had come to a halt, the five bodies were strewn all over the highway. The driver of the other car got out and almost fainted when he saw five bodies sprawled out across the road. Rufus said it took him several minutes to convince the man that he hadn't killed five people.

We started our dissection of our assigned cadaver with the body lying on his stomach. We had to turn him over, and there is nothing as unwieldy as a dead body being turned over on a slab, where one has to be sure that it doesn't fall off. By the time we finished, our lab coats had received another coating of that aromatic preserving fluid. We started on the upper part of the neck and shoulder; Gilbert and I were on one side and the other two students were working on the other. I am sure that this was designed so that we started on an area where we could do as little damage as possible. At the beginning we approached the dissection very tentatively, but when we found out how difficult it really was to do any significant damage, we sped up.

There was more to do than we, with our lack of dissection expertise, could keep up with. In order to not get behind, people began to come in at night to do further dissection. Before long, half the class would be there working after-hours. In due time, people started to bring in food and could be seen eating hamburgers, soft drinks, etc. Perhaps the preserving fluid did something to our olfactory apparatus or we became immune to the smell, but we had gotten to the point where the odor only bothered us when we got on the elevator and people got off. By the time we had dissected the left side of the neck, shoulders, arm, and hand, our partners on the other side had only gotten to the elbow. The proctors never said a word about it. They allowed you to dig your own hole.

One of this pair was reputed, by himself mostly, to have a master's degree in organic chemistry, with a 4.0 grade-point average. This is the same fellow who had never seen anyone as dead as our cadaver.

My thought was that having a master's degree in organic chemistry should give him an edge up in biochemistry. It so happened that our first exam of the year was in biochemistry. We took the exam one morning, and after it was over, I felt as if I had done well.

But in the conclave that always occured in the hallway after an exam, people were roaming around talking and saying such things as, "What did you put on such and such . . .?" Our friend was free with the answers that he gave to many of the exam questions. They weren't anywhere close to my answers. I decided that I was in way over my head, and I had failed the exam. The next day, the tests had been graded and returned. We went to our one-hour lecture and afterward proceeded to the lab where our test results were located. When the questions for the exam were given out, our answers were written in a blue book. These were small booklets with blank lined pages and covered with blue paper. In biochemistry your blue book was placed face down at your lab space. When I got there, it was lying on the lab bench face down. I stared at it for a while and finally summoned enough courage to look. Fully expecting a failing grade, I picked it up, flipped it over, and looked at a ninety-six.

In biochemistry, when you were studying chemical effects in the body, you used your own body as a source of scientific raw material to study. For instance, when studying gastric juice, one of your less sadistic (you hope) classmates would pass a gastric tube down your throat and into your stomach and aspirate some gastric juice for chemical analysis. Of course, those of us with sensitive gag reflexes wound up putting their gastric juice all over the lab floor. The entire lab was filled with students sitting on stools with their faces beet red, their eyes bulging, and gastric juice drooling out the side of their mouths around an inserted gastric tube. We would learn later that if one inserts the nasogastric tube through the nose, there is much less gag reflex elicited.

When studying the role of diet on the excretion of chemicals in urine, we had to carry around a big jug to collect a twenty-four-hour urine sample for analysis of our urine. This was after being on a diet rich in various things such as salt and purines, the building blocks for nucleic acids, DNA, RNA, and so forth. We had become wise by then. We collected the urine, but went up the hill to a diner and poured a shaker full of salt in it. The lab proctor said that he had never seen that much salt excreted before. He was ecstatic.

Our next big test was gross anatomy. This, if you recall, was the grim reaper course that separated the wheat from the chaff. There was really a preponderance of gloomy faces as we stood outside the gross lab waiting for the doors to be opened. Upon entering, you were handed a sheet of paper with numbers going down the left side. Each number represented a corresponding tag number attached to an anatomical entity on the cadavers. On these tags, which might be looped around a nerve, blood vessel, or attached to a particular muscle, were specific questions regarding each tagged specimen.

There would be written on the tag questions such as, "What is the name of this vessel, what is its origin, what organ does it supply, etc., ?" or, "What muscle is this, what is its origin, what is its insertion, what arteries and veins supply it, and what nerve innervates it?" You would then write your answers next to the corresponding number on the answer sheet. After an interval of so many minutes, time would be called and everyone would move to the other side, or the next tank, to repeat the process. This was repeated over and over until everyone had rotated through both sides of each cadaver.

When it was over, I felt as if a three hundred pound weight had been lifted off my shoulders. There wasn't a single question on that exam that I couldn't answer. I had met the big monster head on, and I won. A few others and I felt so good that we walked across 20th Street to a diner, and I bought myself a cup of coffee just completely relaxed. I knew I was going to make it. John T. and I celebrated by going to Britling's Cafeteria that night.

Sometime during the fall, the school announced that each class had to elect a slate of class officers for some reason or other. I don't know who did it, but someone put my name up for class president, and I won. I sort of figured that the older guys felt I was young enough to be impressed with the fact I had been elected class president. It definitely didn't go to my head. The same thing happened again the next year, and I was president during my sophomore year.

The only thing I ever had to do involved panty raids. Back in the fifties, there was a fad of boys making raids on girls' dormitories and stealing panties--really a very childish thing to do. But whoever claimed that sophomore males were staid individuals? At the very end of our sophomore year, a couple of guys came to tell me that the Dean was looking for me. I went to his office, and he practically shouted, "We have a report that some medical students are planning a panty raid on the student nurses' dormitory. You must contact your classmates and tell them that we will not condone such behavior."

I just stood there for a second or two, and then I replied, "These students in my class are grown men and have just finished fighting a war. You don't really think that they would do anything so childish, do you?"

He replied, "I don't know, but you need to tell them that we will not tolerate such a thing."

I said, "Yes, sir," and I left the office and went back to my room. There was no raid.

During the ensuing months there was a monotonous nature to each day. We would arise before dawn, trudge down to the fast food bar, grab a doughnut and a cup of coffee, and go to class. We would have a biochemistry lecture and lab, then a micro anatomy lecture and lab in the mornings, and then we would have a gross anatomy lecture and lab in the afternoon. I finally figured the strategy of this monotony. They were teaching us what went on in the human body chemically and what the microscopic anatomy was of the large items that we were studying in gross anatomy.

We would get up in the dark, and when we got out of gross lab it was dark, and we smelled bad again. On the weekends, I would catch a city bus to the Birmingham bus station, get a ticket to Gadsden and ride to its bus station. From there, I would walk to Nancy's and my apartment, which was about five or six blocks away. After spending the weekend with Nancy, I would get up Monday morning at 4:00 a.m., walk to the city bus stop, and catch a bus out to Attalla, Alabama, where I would catch a train to Birmingham. Before the train would have left the station, I would have settled in a seat and put my ticket where the conductor could see it and cancel it. In those days the conductor carried a small instrument that allowed him to punch a round hole in your ticket so it couldn't be used again. Soon I would be sound asleep.

I would be awakened by the conductor calling, "Birmingham, Birmingham. Next stop, Birmingham!" After just a few rides, he knew my face and would make sure that I was awake. I would disembark, walk down to 20th Street, and catch a bus to the school. I would stop by my room, drop off my bag, stop by the food bar, rapidly gulp a cup of coffee and my usual doughnut, and I would be settled in my seat for the eight o'clock lecture. This went on all year.

At the end of the semester, we had finished biochemistry and micro anatomy. We would continue gross anatomy and start physiology the second semester.

The assistant dean called in our friend from Sewanee since he had not passed a single exam all year. They explained to him that they did not want to see him fail and also explained that the state of Alabama had a lot of money invested in him from the previous semester. If he would apply himself more diligently the coming semester and pass all of his exams, they would allow him to attend another school during the summer, such as Michigan, and make up the courses he had just finished.

He was really a very nice guy and was always pleasant, hospitable, and seemed to not have a care in the world. He accepted the conditions, and off we went into the second semester. He did set a record. As of that time, he was the only student who never passed an exam in an entire year. They notified Sewanee that he had failed and they replied, "How did he get in?" It turned out that he had worked in the registrar's office, and when it came time to submit a transcript of his grades he furnished them with an enviable record. It was all totally false.

Through the years since then, I have thought about his reason for doing this. I think he may have started out with the intention to graduate from medical school—a real con. However, as the year went along and it became obvious that he wasn't going to be able to pull it off, I think that he was just seeing how long he could ride the scam. He was never worried about his obvious plight, he studied less than any of us, and when he was dismissed he acted, "Oh well, it was fun while it lasted." I was irritated with him about one this in this entire affair: He took the place of a viable candidate for his slot in our class. He cheated someone out of the chance to be a physician so he could play this little game. I have no idea what happened to him.

Physiology was added in place of biochemistry and microbiology this semester. We continued to dissect our cadaver, and at the end of the semester we took the brain that we had removed earlier in the year, and studied neuroanatomy. At the end of that course, I could trace origins of nerves from the tiniest portion of the central neural system to its innervation of some far away organ. Unfortunately, I can't do it anymore, but I can still do a lot of it. It comes in very handy when trying to figure out what is wrong with a patient with neurological complaints.

That summer, I worked at Fort McClellan just outside Anniston, Alabama, and only about nine miles from Jacksonville. Since

Nancy's teaching job had also ended, we moved in with her parents in Jacksonville. I now was working and getting a journeyman's wages, so life was good. They were renovating a portion of the fort so that the WAC headquarters could be transferred there. I spent my time redoing the plumbing in the kitchens of the mess halls.

The important thing that happened as a result of this job was that I was able to buy my first car. I bought it from a co-worker at a reasonable price of about twelve hundred dollars. If that sounds cheap, you should know that a similar new car would have cost thirty-five hundred dollars. It was a slant-back black Chevrolet; what year it was, I don't remember. It was clean and had good tires, the engine ran well, and gas was only twenty-five cents a gallon. I don't know if it was an advantage or not, but it burned just enough oil that I had to add a quart every few hundred miles. It was sort of a self-oil-changing arrangement. Now there would be no more riding buses, catching trains, or waiting for a city bus in freezing cold at an unlit stop in the dark before sunup.

Nancy was unable to get a job teaching in the Birmingham area again this year, and she had to accept a job in a country school outside Jacksonville. I packed my belongings in my new (to me) car and drove to school. I moved back into my room with a new roommate and started my sophomore season. This year was devoted mostly to learning about diseases and their effects on the body (pathology), learning about things that cause disease (microbiology), how to diagnose them (clinical pathology), and how to treat them (pharmacology).

By now the school had built a basic science building across the street from the hospital that contained all the teaching labs needed for the students' labs and research labs for the faculty. In addition, it contained the Dental School, which used the same courses, and also a dental clinic. Dr. Joe Volker had been enticed down from his position of dean of the School of Dentistry at Tufts University to start a new dental school in Alabama. He brought a lot of his own personnel down with him from Tufts. He required that all of his dental faculty have double degrees. His clinical faculty was required to have a degree not only in dentistry, but also an MD degree. Therefore, in the second year we began to see some of these individuals in our clinical classes. Later, they would go through some of our clinical rotations that were not covered in their dental program.

This group included a young, blond-headed chief of oral surgery named "Scotty" McCallum who would go on to be my roommate when we were house officers became, in this order, dean of the dental school, vice president of the medical center, and eventually, president of the University of Alabama in Birmingham. You can see what a good influence I had on him when we were roommates!

The university used land that it already owned to build this building. I would discover much later in my career that the university was one of biggest land owners in Jefferson County. This particular plot of land was the property of the athletic department. A school never knows when it might need to build a football field across the street from the hospital. At the eastern end of the building, an extension was added that ran across the entire dental building. This housed the extension service of the university, which offered courses mainly at the freshman and sophomore levels. Ultimately, this would grow into the University of Alabama at Birmingham. It also housed a small space for the fledgling services of the Alabama Public Services TV station.

We now had regular lecture halls, good labs, and enough space to spread out a little. We also began having an hour lecture in psychiatry once a week. This was to continue throughout the remainder of our schooling until graduation. What I got from this is that a psychiatric diagnosis is purely the personal opinion of the person making the diagnosis. There is absolutely no scientific way to make an ironclad, provable diagnosis. In fact, many years ago, the chairman of the Department of Psychiatry at Tulane University made a discovery that the spinal fluid of schizophrenic patients contained an abnormal protein. Instead of hailing this as a major observation, the American Psychiatry Association tried to have him kicked out. Now that is really scientific behavior: don't bother me with the facts—I have my mind made up.

In microbiology, we studied the various bacteria and viruses that caused illnesses and learned to grow and identify pathologic bacteria. In pharmacology, we studied the different classes of drugs, how they acted, and demonstrated that in the laboratories. One thing that I particularly remember is one of the instructors saying, "I love hydrogen peroxide; it looks like it is trying so hard."

In clinical pathology, we were taught how to do various clinical tests, such as urinalysis, CBC's (complete blood counts), and so forth. As before, we used our own body fluids for the various tests. One day we were taught how to make a blood smear on a microscope slide and how to stain it. When we began to look at it, we had to learn how to identify the various blood cells and evaluate the number of platelets, red cells, etc. Suddenly, we noted all the professors were all huddled around Rawls Lindsey's microscope. He had made a diagnosis of chronic myelogenous leukemia on himself. He finished school, served his internship, and practiced in North Mobile County for a few scant years before succumbing to the disease.

This year seemed to go by much faster than the freshman year did. Maybe it was because we didn't feel as much pressure on us. That summer, I had my last plumbing job in Childersburg, Alabama, building an addition on a rayon plant. I was working for Pap again, as he was superintendent of the project. I really was working as a steamfitter, and Tom was working as a welder. We got the usual lecture that we would be watched by the other men, and we would need to work harder than anyone so that there could be no charge of favoritism from any of our co-workers. As far as I know there wasn't.

Nancy and I rented a two-room apartment in the home of a very nice old lady, and Pap and Mama rented one across and down the street in Sylacauga, Alabama, about ten miles away from the job. When we moved in and paid our rent in advance for the coming month, we were essentially broke until payday the next day. However, at the moment we only had a little over a dollar in cash and no groceries. Of course, we could have gone to my parents for help, but our pride wouldn't let us do that. We walked down to a small market and found a box of spaghetti, with accompanying sauce, for a little under a dollar. It was a fairly large box, and we cooked the whole thing. I suppose that it was because we didn't have anything else to eat, or we were just so grateful to have something to eat, that we ate the entire thing. We both had stomachaches afterward.

We gave up on getting Nancy a teaching job, but that wasn't a sad decision since, if I may put it delicately, she absolutely despised teaching. On the suggestion of a classmate's wife, she interviewed for a job in the actuarial department of Protective Life Insurance Company. To make a long story short she got the job, which paid more than teaching. She would work there for many years until we had to leave to enter the Air Force. Protective Life would continue to play a role in our lives, however, as we shall see later. We found an apartment building where some of the other medical students lived, and with some of the money that I earned through the summer, we bought a fourteen-inch TV set with its own stand. We placed it in our not-so-majestic living room, spread our rabbit ears antenna, and declared ourselves ready for the coming academic year.

My third year was the beginning of the clinical years. One half of the class would spend one semester in internal medicine, and the other half would spend one semester in surgery. At the midyear we would swap. I started on the medicine wards. There was a strict dress code. Students were to wear white pants and a white jacket. The preferred dress was an intern's jacket that buttoned up to the neck and had the student's name stitched in red over the left pocket. Students could never, I repeat never, appear on the ward in scrubs.

There were essentially twenty-five students on medicine and twenty-five students on surgery. On the services, we would be further subdivided into groups of five, with each group being assigned to a particular ward. On the ward, each student was assigned certain patients that were there when we arrived, and subsequent admissions would be assigned to the next individuals who were up for a new patient. When assigned a patient, it meant taking total responsibility for that patient's care. If he or she needed a procedure done, it was done under supervision. If simple lab work such as urinalysis or blood work was required, the student collected and did the laboratory work in a lab provided for the students on the sixth floor. You were supposed to have learned how to do that in clinical pathology. If your patient was to be presented at conference or on rounds, you did it.

If you were presenting to Dr. Harrison, there were two things you needed to remember. The first was that you had better be acutely aware of the difference between "lie" and "lay." This was one of his pet peeves, using these words incorrectly. He would stop one's presentation and explain the difference between "lie" and "lay." It was evident to him that a physician should be able to get that correct. The other thing was never to speak of a patient as a case of some sort of malady. This always sent him into orbit. He would explain cryptically that a patient is not a case of anything, but is a patient with some malady. One such episode was all that was needed to make everyone acutely aware of that simple fact. It was constantly drummed into us that our patient came first, and the care of that patient took precedence over everything that might need doing. No matter if you had a conference or a lecture, you were automatically excused if your patient needed you. This was the way that it was impressed upon us that nothing came before our patient's care and welfare.

All of these patients were on the indigent service, which meant that they were housed on floors with eight- to ten-bed wards. All of the beds were capable of being curtained off into a private setting if it were needed. Hospitalization in ward beds was a cost-saving move for it required fewer nurses to provide nursing care than if each patient was cordoned off in a private room somewhere. These patients were provided nursing care not only by the floor nurses, but also by junior and senior nursing students and the medical student that was assigned to that patient.

The physician's care was provided by the resident physicians and the interns assigned to that floor and those wards. These physicians were, in turn, supervised by a faculty member who was also assigned to those same wards on a rotational basis, and he or she made work rounds every morning with the house staff. In addition, the chief of staff of medicine or surgery made weekly teaching rounds. Laboratory costs were kept to a minimum, for the medical students performed those duties also, except for the more complicated lab procedures.

Prior to admission, each patient received a financial screening and his or her ability to pay was determined. Charges were not made individually to a patient, but an average cost was calculated from the yearly combined costs of all the indigent patients admitted during the past fiscal year, and this total was calculated as an average daily cost (per diem rate) for any and all hospitalized indigent patients. The final cost of a patient's hospital stay was determined by the number of hospital days, multiplied by the per diem rate. Jefferson County, or another participating county, was then billed for that amount of money. If a patient were rated as being able to pay a certain percentage of that cost, then that would be billed to that patient, and a length of time was set according to the ability of the patient's family to pay a monthly payment. In this manner, all indigent patients of Jefferson County received better than average hospital care and at a much lower cost.

During our hospital teaching programs, lectures were given each day at noon from ancillary departments such as dermatology and obstetrics. I remember vividly a lecture in obstetrics by Dr. James Garber. He was a white-headed little man with a small tolerance for stupid questions. One day he was lecturing on delivery of a baby by version and extraction. In those days, if a mother was not making progress in her labor, or the baby was not progressing in coming on down the vaginal canal, the doctor would perform a version and extraction. In this procedure, the physician would don a sterile version glove, which reached up a small distance above the elbow, and he would reach up into the uterus, grab the baby's feet, and gently turn the baby around, delivering the baby feet-first (breach delivery). He spoke about how sometimes when your arm was in the uterus, there would be a uterine contraction, and your arm would become numb from the pressure. One of my classmates raised his hand and said, "Now, understand Dr. Garber, I wouldn't mind doing it, but is there any danger that your arm might be permanently damaged?"

Without missing a beat Dr. Garber replied, "No, V——, there are no teeth in there."

Every Saturday was show time. First, there was a CPC (clinical pathology conference). This was run by the pathology department and consisted of the presentation of a patient who had died and had received an autopsy. This was done by an oral and a written summary of the patient's history, physical examination, and laboratory work. Someone from a clinical department would discuss the clinical and laboratory findings and give his diagnosis, along with his reasons. The autopsy findings were then presented, and the real diagnosis was shown. It was always something that was way off the wall, and there was no clue to lead one to the proper diagnosis. Seldom did anyone get it right, a fact that gave me great comfort when I would also miss them later on in my life. It also stressed the fact that the brightest of physicians could not always make the right diagnosis. It kept us humble.

This was followed by the medical-surgical conference held by Dr. Harrison and Dr. Lyons. Here, a patient would be presented who was currently a patient in the hospital. Following this, there was a rousing discussion with a great deal of repartee, all in good humor, but also superlative in its teaching. Dr. Lyons was a pompous soul who would pontificate with his entire egotistical splendor on the surgeon's role in the care of the patient. Dr. Harrison would respond with rapier-like wit and insight. He would embellish this with cutting barbs such as, "I am going to take off one these weekends and learn to be a surgeon." The auditorium was always crowded, and everyone was always keenly disappointed if they were unable to attend.

On the wards, when a new patient was assigned to you, you were required to write an admissions note on the patient's chart that detailed his medical history of the present illness, past medical history, review of the patient's body systems, and his or her physical exam. This had to be recorded in longhand according to a small pocket-size book that was distributed to every student on day one. You would ask all the questions, including those that included his or her sex life and document all the positive things that pertained to this particular illness. It always embarrassed me to ask someone about his or her sex life. I had been raised as a child never to ask personal questions. In the review of the various body systems, you would have to write down all the things you asked the patient about. This included all the facts that pertained to the patient's illness, but also the things that the patient didn't have, such as there was no shortness of breath, orthopnea, cough, etc., etc.

By the time the semester ended, everyone knew that little book and could recite it verbatim. I still can for that matter. At the end of the write up you were required to write down your impression of the diagnosis, followed by a list of differential diagnoses. You then wrote down what supported your impression from data acquired from the history and physical, and then what laboratory work was needed to rule in or out your differential diagnoses. Dr. Harrison would become very irritated if you suggested laboratory work that was really not needed. If you suggested something that wasn't needed, he would suggest that you were guessing and would hope that something would be abnormal so as to give you a clue. This rule is not followed presently, as physicians order laboratory work to cover questions which may be asked in a malpractice law suit. Each one knows they are not needed, but it is a matter of protection of one's back. Unfortunately, this practice does undeniably run up medical care costs.

Assigned to a medical ward were a medical resident, one or two interns (MDs in their first year of training after graduation), and a chief medical resident who was over all the medical residents. There was no extra house staff stuck off in reserve. About two months into the semester, our intern, Dr. George Blue Penton, became ill. He was the only intern assigned to our ward, so there was a minor crisis with a house staff member shortage. Dr. Harrison solved it by declaring that one of the junior medical students on that particular service would serve as acting intern until Dr. Penton returned.

I don't know who decided who it would be, but I was notified that for the next week or so I was going to be the official intern on the ward. This was not particularly an honor, but it was a chance to learn something not ordinarily offered. In this position I was required to work every other night, and I was the one the nurses called when something went wrong with a patient. I don't mean to suggest that I was Mr. Cool about this whole thing. You have to remember that I was a junior student with about two months' exposure to internal medicine under my belt. I read as much as I had time for, and I was assured that it was all right to call the resident when I was uncertain what to do. I didn't say it, but I thought that meant that I would probably keep him on the phone all night. This lasted about a week, and George Blue came back to work. I went back to being a regular junior student again.

About two weeks later, another intern on another medical ward became sick. The chief resident came down and told me that Dr. Harrison wanted me to step in as an intern on that ward. This endeared me to everyone but my classmates on that particular ward. They told me they could handle it, and one of their group should be acting intern. I told them that I was just doing what I was told to do, but if they felt sufficiently slighted they could take their complaints to the chief resident. I heard nothing else about it, and this tenure as an intern was a lot easier than the first.

We didn't have any recurrences of an ill intern for the rest of the semester. There was one good thing that came out of it—Dr. Harrison could put my name and my face together. Toward the end of the academic year, he called me into his office and wanted me to drop out of school for a year and work with him. I don't think I have ever had an offer that flattered me like that. It would have been a dream come true, but as I told him, if I dropped out of school for a year I would be drafted as a buck private in the rear ranks. In my later life he would step in and give some moral and practical support.

Before leaving medicine and Dr. Harrison, I need to add one anecdote that perfectly typifies Dr. Harrison and his dedication to teaching and patient care. In his later years, Dr. Harrison moved down to Alexander City, Alabama, where he would have students come work with him in teaching clinics that he had set up in the local community hospital. This was after I had returned and was on the faculty. We got word that Dr. Harrison had experienced a coronary occlusion, but he was resting comfortably. Joe Reeves, one of his protégés and friend, immediately set out for Alexander City. When he got there, he entered Dr. Harrison's room and found him sitting up in bed with a tape recorder. He said, "Quickly, Joe, we've got to get our description of coronary pain changed. It's not at all like we have been describing it."

At the end of the semester, I switched to the surgery rotation. I was looking forward to this rotation because I was fairly adept with my hands, and I assumed that I was going to enjoy that aspect of medicine. I was horribly disappointed in this expectation. It was mainly dull repetition of procedures. I got no joy in scrubbing up, going into the operating room, being gloved and gowned, standing at the far end of the operating table, and holding a retractor. One has to understand that in an operation, no one can see a blessed thing except the operator, his or her first assistant, and perhaps the scrub nurse.

A lot of my classmates were gung ho about all of this and were constantly going around with a long piece of cord, which they would loop around a chair back and start practicing tying knots. I began to understand why Dr. Harrison would say, "There are two kinds of doctors. There are thinkers and doers, and the doers make surgeons."

I did have one experience in the surgery rotation that was very interesting. This was a fellow about thirty years of age who had rheumatic fever as a child. As it so often does, it attacked the mitral valve of his heart and left the patient with a scarred valve that had partially calcified. The mitral valve is situated between the left atrium (the upper chamber of the heart) and the left ventricle, and anything that interferes with the flow of blood between the two chambers has drastic results. First, if the blood cannot flow freely into the left ventricle, it will begin to back up and cause pulmonary hypertension (high blood pressure). Because the blood doesn't flow into the left ventricle, when the ventricle contracts there is very little blood ejected into the body. This leads to decreased blood flow to the brain, etc., and the patient becomes incapacitated.

Heart surgery was in its infancy in those days, and to fix this fellow was going to require open heart surgery. This was long before cardiac bypass machines. The procedure at that time was to open the left side of the chest and make an incision through the wall of the left atrium. After that small area had been clamped off with a large hemostat. The surgeon, wearing two gloves on his hand, would stick his finger through the incision site where it was tied in place by a pucker draw string that prevented any leakage of blood around the inserted finger when the atrium contracted. By feel alone, the surgeon examined the valve and determined if it seemed feasible to just crack open the valve with the inserted finger. If not, then a small lancet, which had been secured on the index finger of the surgeon between the two sets of rubber gloves, was pushed out through the tip of the exterior glove so that it was fully exposed in the beating left atrium. The surgeon then inserted the blade into the valve opening and sliced the scarred valve tissue along the natural opening line, thus freeing up the mitral valve opening to open and close again. All this was done blindly.

When the valve was obviously opening and closing as well as it was going to, the surgeon withdrew his finger and the pucker string was drawn closed to seal the atrial wall. This fellow was my patient just by the luck of the draw. When he was taken to surgery, everybody and his uncle was in the operating room to see the first open heart surgery in the state. Because he was my patient, I was at my usual spot at the end of the table, and a lot of the bigwigs were stationed around the wall. Fortunately, the operation went smooth as silk. When it was over, Dr. Lyons stepped back, stripped off his gloves, and said, "Line them up, Tinsley."

There were more mild clashes between the surgery residents and the medical students than there were in medicine. There truly is such a thing as the surgical personality, a need to show everyone who is in charge, sometimes to a fault. I recall an occurrence with a friend of mine who was an older student, being a veteran of the Pacific Theater. His patient had been to surgery that day, and the surgery resident told him that he wanted him to sit with the patient all night and check vital signs every thirty minutes. Well, there was nothing that really called for that to be done. It was just the surgical personality coming out, showing who was in charge. So that night, John would call the resident every thirty minutes to tell him what the vital signs were, explaining that since he was so concerned about them he wanted to keep him informed. About one o'clock in the morning the resident realized he was being outsmarted, and he told John to discontinue the vital signs. Incidentally, John became a surgeon.

Sometimes the clashes between surgical personalities would have serious repercussions. One day Dr. Lyons and his chief resident were operating together on one of Dr. Lyons's patients. Dr. Lyons was being more belligerent than usual that day, and he began to berate the poor resident at every little turn. The hapless resident could only sit there and absorb the verbal abuse. Finally he had all that he could bear, and he stepped back, stripped off his gloves, and shouted, "Dr. Lyons, you have cancer of the soul." With that he stormed out, turned in his resignation, and transferred to another surgical program. It is considered bad taste to run off one's chief resident.

Here is one more anecdote about Dr. Lyons, who was a source of terror for the medical students, a role in which he reveled. One of my friends in the class ahead of me was scheduled to scrub on one of his patients, who happened to be Dr. Lyons's patient. He scrubbed up for the operation after his academic betters had finished. He entered the operating room after everyone else had already been gowned and gloved. The scrub nurse came over with my friend's gown and inquired, "What size glove do you wear, doctor?" No one had ever asked him that before. His mind went blank and he could only think of the size work glove he used at home in his garden.

He stammered, "Uh, size nine." Now, size eight is a large glove and it is rarely required.

The nurse said, "Oh."

Dr. Lyons looked around and said, "Damn." They found him some size nine gloves and put them on his hands. His fingers only reached about three fourths of the way to the end of the gloves' fingers, and the body of the glove hung loosely off of his hands. He trudged over to the operating table with his floppy gloves and the empty fingers flopping around. Dr. Lyons never said a word, but the resident said he could see the twinkle in his eye.

We finished our junior year unscathed. We still had all of our classmates with whom we finished the sophomore year. That summer I had lab jobs, etc., and my summers of physical labor were over.

The senior year was our exposure to actual obstetrics, not just lectures. We were scheduled to have two rotations of obstetrics this year, a month of in-hospital deliveries, and a month of home deliveries. They offered the in-house delivery to any seniors who wanted to take the course for a month in August. This was reputed to be a hellish month, so four of us decided we were going to take it and get it over with. The course ran for one month, and after a short introduction of two or three days of lectures, we literally moved into the hospital.

We would not be allowed out for thirty days. The only time one could see his family was their coming over to eat with him in the hospital cafeteria. This, of course, was predicated on the fact that one didn't have a patient with impending delivery or was not tied up in a delivery. The delivery area for the black patients consisted of two delivery rooms separated by a scrub area and a large labor ward that held about twenty beds. At the end of the labor ward was a door that opened into a small room containing some cabinets, a sink, and a hot plate. Thus, we were given all the amenities that a medical student needed: a bathroom adjoined the "kitchen." A door was located in the "kitchen" on the opposite wall from the labor room door which opened up into our palatial sleeping quarters. This consisted of eight beds, four on each side, and a bed light for reading about obstetrics in bed. I came to hate this place.

The intention was to get one as much practical experience as possible in a short time frame and to give us the necessary academic knowledge as well. To accomplish this, the four of us took care of every charity delivery that was admitted that month. I haven't described the facilities for the white charity patients because there weren't any admitted during that month. Also, the dress code was altered for this course. We ate, slept, and worked in scrubs, often for a couple of days at a time in the same suit. When one becomes sleep deprived, it is difficult to remember what occurred when.

We attended obstetrics clinic in the morning, except weekends. We examined pregnant women at all stages of pregnancy to insure good health and to prevent premature births. When clinic was over, we returned to the delivery area to see any new patients and check on the ones in labor. When a patient was admitted, she was assigned to one of us according to a rotational schedule. We stayed close to our patient until she delivered her offspring under the supervision of a resident in obstetrics. We learned to monitor the progress of the labor by doing rectal exams periodically.

When a woman goes into labor and the baby starts to slowly migrate down the birth canal, the doctor can feel the baby's head and the uterine cervix by doing a rectal exam. As the labor progresses, the cervix opening starts to thin and begins to be thinner and thinner as the baby's head begins to enlarge the cervical opening by simple brute force. When the cervix is completely effaced (i.e. fully dilated), that is the time to take the patient to the delivery table. There would be times when multiple patients of a student would be in labor at the same time, leaving him very little time for rest. Many times during that month one of us would be working in his sleep. I distinctly remember going to sleep standing up at the delivery table. It was only for a brief moment, and I didn't fall to the floor. I may be kin to a horse since they can sleep standing up.

There were moments of levity to lighten the load, however. There was the time I walked by Andy Hagen examining a patient in labor, only to discover that he had fallen asleep with his bald head lying on the woman's fully pregnant belly and with his index finger in her rectum. Then there was the time Andy Anderson sneaked out of the hospital one night, drove down to a produce market, and returned with a large sack full of green peanuts still on the vine. We scrounged up a pot from somewhere, picked the green peanuts off the vines, and boiled them in salty water. We ate them while they were still warm. It was a meal truly fit for a king.

Then there was the time Andy Hagen asked the chief resident if he could get off long enough to get a haircut. Of course, he was bald (his nickname was Dermal Dome) and had only a fringe of black hair encircling the lower aspects of his skull. The resident said that he supposed that it would be all right and Andy replied, "I always get my hair cut in Sylacauga." This was where his family lived, about sixty miles to the southeast.

The postpartum ward was down the hall from the labor and delivery area, and all of the young mothers were placed there to assure there were no postpartum complications. We had women of all ages in that ward. We had girls from the age of twelve up to women in their forties. The young girls would say that they wanted to have their children when they were young so they could enjoy them. Practically, what happened was that the maternal grandmother would raise the child, and they would call them their "yard children."

All of these young girls wanted fancy names for their babies and would not accept the popular names suggested by us. We became inventive, so now there are a lot of adults walking around with names such as Terramycin, Achromycin, etc. My favorite of all the names were a pair of twins named El Paso and El Toro Sludge. I did have a patient brought in whose name was Fragile (pronounced fra-gi-lee). I said to the father, "That is an interesting name; where did you get it?"

He replied, "Off a box."

I delivered approximately sixty babies that month, which was enough for me to realize I didn't want to do that for the remainder of my medical career. I have never regretted that decision. When my tour ended, it felt as if I had been released from some sort of incarceration. We went to see the movie *Shane* that night. I don't know whether it was because I was free or not, but I thought it was one of the best movies I had ever seen.

We had a month's rotation through gynecology, which was under the supervision of Dr. Nick Jones. When Dr. Garber retired in a few years, the two departments were merged under Dr. Jones. He was a delightful man who reveled in being a professional country boy. I remember being on rounds when the residents presented a patient and gave Dr. Jones a differential diagnosis of four things. Dr. Jones put his hands in his pants pockets, rocked back on his heels, and said, "Now boys, when you give me a differential diagnosis of four things, you've pretty well taken the middle out of the book." Gynecology was all right, but it was like surgery—in a very limited area.

Home delivery was an interesting experience. These patients were carefully screened, and were multiparous (many pregnancies) mothers who usually had delivered five or six children, and without any sort of difficulty with this current pregnancy. Andy Anderson and I were partners in this endeavor. We had a home delivery kit that was loaded into the same van in which Rufus had his cadaver experience, along with a stretcher, on the outside chance that we would need to transport the patient to the hospital for some reason. On our first trip, we arrived at a small house and were let into a tiny living room. There were people everywhere. There seemed to be a multitude of small children along with older aunts, uncles, and grandparents, too. There may have been a few neighbors thrown in there also.

When we entered the small bedroom off of the living room, the mother was lying in bed and there were children of seemingly every age sitting, standing, lying, and slithering around on the floor. I have no idea whether they were all hers or not. We finally got all of the kids out and proceeded to examine the mother. It did not take long to decide that this was false labor and that she was not ready for delivery. She was mortified for having called us out too early. We assured her that it was perfectly all right, and it was better to call us than to wait too long. We packed up and left.

About three or four nights later, we got a call to return. We knew the way this time, and we arrived shortly after being called. There were only a few people there this trip, and when we went into the bedroom there were only five or six children. We shooed the children out and pulled back the covers on the bed. There, lying between his mother's legs, was a little boy, calmly sucking on his thumb. The mother said, "I wanted to make sure the time was right before calling you again. I didn't have no trouble birthing him."

Medical schools these days don't offer courses like our in-patient and home delivery anymore. In a way it is a shame, because what are these physicians going to tell their offspring about their obstetrics experiences? On another note, Andy Hagen wound up going into Ob-Gyn. as a profession, despite his experiences.

We had one rotation through the medical clinics such as hematology, outpatient internal medicine, and neurology. I had an experience in neurology that I recall with some remorse. A young black man came in for a routine visit as follow up to control his grand mal seizures (epilepsy). Seizures were sometimes very difficult to control in those days because of the scarcity of any effectual drugs. This was a tall, thin young man—a little younger than I was and who seemed very shy. He had just entered the examining area, and we were both standing by my desk. Suddenly he developed a blank stare on his face, his eyes rolled up in his head, and I, in my youthful ignorance, had no idea what was going on. He fell straight forward before I could think to catch him, and he landed with the sickening sound of his face striking directly on the concrete floor. Of course, he was having a seizure.

We rolled him over, kept him from chewing his tongue, and waited for the seizure to end. While he was in his post-convulsive state, we cleaned and bandaged his severely abraded face. I have always felt guilty that I didn't know enough to prevent him from falling and doing damage to himself. When he recovered, he left the clinic with a look of shame on his face for what had occurred. Perhaps I shared that shame somewhat for being unable to do more to relieve him. People with epilepsy in those days were regarded as outcasts of society. Preachers railed against them as being possessed by the devil, people shunned them for their behavior, and it was very difficult for the severe ones to obtain employment. It is not so different today about some other deviations from "normal" that some people have to cope with daily.

My other rotation was pediatrics. After my experiences with

older people who kept breaking something else after the physician had just finished fixing another problem, Pediatrics was a godsend. Infants would be brought in with some type of dysentery, which caused them to become frightfully dehydrated from loss of fluids and electrolytes through their profuse diarrhea. On admission, they literally looked like prunes because of dehydration. They would be in severe acidosis, but after a night of the proper amount of IV fluids and electrolytes, the next morning they were perfectly normal in appearance. It certainly helped to have basically healthy tissue to try to heal. However, I still thought that I would like to go into internal medicine or general practice.

In those days the twelfth floor of the hospital contained medicine beds, and at the end of a long corridor was the infectious disease ward. Here were housed the people who had contagious diseases, the majority of which were usually pediatrics. In those days we had a lot of meningitis, poliomyelitis, diphtheria, etc. When I was on pediatrics, some of my patients were housed in that unit. In order to get there, I had to walk through a medical ward. I remember walking down that corridor and looking at the medicine patients as I walked by. In one room was a patient in kidney failure, with uremic "frost" on his lips; another housed a comatose patient who had suffered from a stroke, with his head turned to the side and breathing with the gurgling sounds that patients with a stroke so often make. Another room contained a patient who was a diabetic, in coma with gangrene of both feet. I looked at these poor souls. I thought of the vibrant protoplasm I was working with in pediatrics, and I said to myself, "I can't do this sort of practice the remainder of my life." I decided right then that I was going into pediatrics. I have never, ever regretted that decision.

As the end of the senior year neared we had to start thinking of internships. In order to get a state medical license to practice, physicians were required to have finished medical school and a year of internship. At one time, the requirement read a rotating internship, which meant rotating through all the services for two months each. This was intended to prepare the doctor for general practice, but now people were beginning to specialize in only one field of medicine and programs were beginning to offer straight internships. This meant no rotations to a different service anytime in the internship, unless it was a prescribed part of the training period.

The University of Alabama Hospital was offering a straight

internship in pediatrics for the first time. It would incorporate time spent at the Children's Hospital, a small private hospital located a few blocks away from University Hospital. There had always been a strained relationship between the private pediatric care in the city and that of the university. This was to be an effort to bring the two programs into harmony. In addition, Children's Hospital would end its residency program, and the University would supply the residents. This was going to greatly increase the teaching material for the residency. I signed up, and I was to be the first and only straight pediatric internship in the program that year.

This would be the first time that I found myself to be the inaugural person in a new endeavor. I believe that I was the only straight intern in my class, with the rest choosing rotating internships. I received a lot of criticism for my selection from my classmates, but I looked at it this way: Why would I want to spend ten months of my internship in programs that I was not going to do, and only months in the program that I was going to do? Now rotating internships are not chosen that much, and if chosen, these interns are treated as red-headed stepkids.

Another new thing was instituted for the graduation ceremony. This year, we were required to participate in the graduation ceremony of the entire university on the main campus. There was a great deal of griping and threats not to go. The answer to that was that we would not receive our diploma unless we attended the ceremony. Now that they explained it that way, we all were glad to accept the invitation. My folks enjoyed the ceremony, the reception at the university president's mansion, and all the other festivities. Luckily, the School of Medicine was the first diplomas presented, and Bentley was one of the first in line. Jimmy Angelich, the oldest graduate, was first. He played halfback on the football team with Bear Bryant, Dixie Howell, and Don Hudson. The newspapers called him "The Angel."

The folks could see in the program that I was in the top ten percent of my class, as I was selected for the Alpha Omega Alpha Honorary Fraternity. I don't know where I ranked in the top ten percent but I know I wasn't first. That clearly belonged to one of the girls in the class, who overwhelmingly led our class all four years. Now I realize that she was a closet lesbian who was found dead in her yard after practicing only a few years in Mobile. It was not officially declared a suicide, I think, in deference to her family, who lived in Mobile. It was a terrible waste of a brilliant mind, but, sadly, a not-too-uncommon ending for closet lesbians at that time.

By the end of the day, I was as tired as after a twenty-four- hour stint on in-patient obstetrics. I rode back with my folks, and I was asleep by the time we reached the city limits of Tuscaloosa. I was now a graduate of the University of Alabama and had just spent my only day on the main campus. I recently attended the fifty-fifth reunion of my medical school class. Everybody was still griping about our having to attend the graduation service on the main campus.

About this time in medical history, the physicians of the land decided there needed to be some program established to help people pay for their hospitalizations. Thus, the insurance company Blue Cross and Blue Shield was established. Blue Cross was created to pay for hospitalization, and Blue Shield was devised to pay for surgery. This was the initial proposal to insure people for hospital care. It was not long before the business interests took control and physicians lost their own management of the innovative proposal to provide payments for health care. Again they were under control of business types whose primary interest was the bottom line. Blue Cross, however, has been loyal to its initial calling and has done as good a job as could be expected under the prevailing circumstances. I understand that they are answerable to their stockholders.

Chapter 6

House Staff Training — Now I Learn to be a Physician

I began my internship at the old Children's Hospital. This was an old three-story red brick building that was still dedicated to wards, a few private rooms, and a policy of parents not being allowed to stay with their children during their hospitalization, except in the few private rooms. It was the place where all of the practicing pediatricians in town hospitalized their patients. In addition, there were programs by state and local programs for specialized services (such as hare lip and cleft palate repairs) which were done under the auspices of State Crippled Children Services, as well as a great deal of charity surgery by various charitable plastic surgeons.

The first floor of the hospital housed the business offices and two large wards. One ward was for infants, and the other one was for children of two years and older. These were used primarily for medical patients, but an occasional patient was admitted for pre-op workups before surgery. On the second floor were patients of all ages who were having a medical workup prior to surgery. An isolation unit was on this floor, along with a small number of private rooms. Another ward was dedicated to post-op patients who were admitted strictly for minor surgery, and they were housed here until they could be safely released home.

Every Thursday, the place would be overrun by children being admitted for tonsillectomy and adenoidectomy. They would be admitted before 7:00 a.m., wheeled up to surgery, have their tonsils and adenoids removed, and be put in this ward to be certain that there were no post-operative complications. It was here that I learned to put postnasal packs in children who were experiencing bleeding from adenoidectomy. Later, we would stop this barbaric custom of wholesale surgical procedures.

The hospital was staffed with extremely competent nurses, many of whom had been employed there for years. In addition, student nurses were assigned to Children's Hospital from some program in Florida, I believe. The nursing staff was accustomed to running the hospital without house staff, except for an occasional resident in their teaching program. They really didn't need house staff to take care of most of the problems that cropped up. In fact, they were very glad to show a green house officer like me the intricacies of everyday patient care, and believe me, I let them do it. Practical learning is not always included in hospital teaching programs. They could start an IV when there was no vein obvious except for a dim blue line on the back of a pudgy little hand of an eight-month-old child.

In addition, my resident was a first-year fellow who had done an anesthesia residency and had had his own general practice for several years. I couldn't have planned a better experience to start off my internship. Dr. Dewey White taught me how to do so many practical things, such as how to easily and properly put in an intradermal skin test, put in a postnasal pack to stem post-adenoidectomy bleeding, endotracheal intubation, one-stitch, venous cutdowns, and many such things. A lot of pediatricians finish their training without acquiring this vital knowledge for the practice of pediatrics. Many pediatricians go to smaller towns to practice and may be the only person in charge. I always told my residents, "In a critical situation, somebody must remain calm and take charge. It had better be you."

After I got my sea legs under me, Dewey and I began to turn our attention to a lot of the private patients who really did not have a definitive diagnosis after a longer than usual hospital stay. These patients would be scrutinized carefully during our leisure moments. Suddenly we began to become aware that a goodly number of these patients had rare diseases. The delicate trick was to reveal our diagnoses without being looked upon as smart-aleck house staff, trying to show up the practicing pediatricians. Somehow we managed to do it, mainly with Dewey leading the way, because he was an older man and respected by the pediatric attending staff. We developed a tiny reputation, and before long, we were covered up with undiagnosed patients being admitted for workups. I began to think that perhaps I was earning my exalted salary of one hundred dollars a month. (The year before, interns had made twenty-five dollars a month).

It wasn't long before I was involved in another first. A disease called kernicterus was relatively common in premature infants in those days. This was a disease caused by the precipitation of a yellow pigment (bilirubin) in the interior central cerebrum of newborn infants. This resulted in their becoming deaf and spastic. A man who later became my friend, Dr. Lou Diamond, had perfected the technique of exchanging twice an infant's total blood volume. This caused a lowering of the blood's bilirubin level and stopped the tearing down of the neonate's red cells from the antibodies that had passed from the mother into the child's blood prior to and during delivery. The exchange of the baby's blood with red cells of a different blood type prevented the continuation of tearing down the red cells. We had admitted a small premature infant with neonatal hemolytic anemia and resulting hyperbilirubinemia. The child was going to need an exchange transfusion to prevent future brain damage.

A newly-arrived pediatrician in town who had just finished his residency at Children's Hospital at Harvard, where Dr. Diamond taught pediatric hematology, had done several exchange transfusions under Dr. Diamond's supervision. It was decided that he and I were going to do an exchange transfusion on the child. Without a lot of hullabaloo, we did an exchange transfusion of twice the baby's blood volume. Everything went well, and both the baby and I survived. It was the first exchange transfusion done in the state of Alabama. These are not done anymore except in rare instances. Hemolytic anemia of the newborn is now prevented, and shining a bilirubin light on the baby controls the elevation of serum bilirubin.

Dr. Diamond and I became good friends later in our lives, when I also had become a hematologist. I once told him about relieving a painful crisis in a sickle-cell anemia patient by a small injection of distilled water in the vein. They didn't have many patients admitted with sickle-cell anemia at Harvard, and a week or so later he called me about treating a patient admitted in a painful sickle-cell anemia crisis. Dr. Diamond was a little leery about giving distilled water IV, since it would cause increased destruction of red cells in a normal person. He was relieved when I reminded him that sickle-cell red cells are very resistant to lowered osmotic surroundings. He told me that he was going to try it and would call me back. He called again in a short while, and he told me that the patient quit hurting before they got the chance to give him the water. I asked, "What do you think happened?"

He replied, "I don't know; maybe we scared it out of him when we told him about the water!"

After my initial rotation, I was transferred to the pediatric service at University Hospital. Although there was a private pediatric service on the fourth floor, essentially all of our patients were admitted to the pediatric service on the third floor and the contagious unit on the twelfth floor. The third floor was for black children, and the fourth floor was for white children, both charity and non-charity. This service was a hotbed of acute care pathology, and there was no letup in the volume of patients that came through. I became very proficient in fluid and electrolyte therapy. In the 1930s, vomiting and diarrhea were the leading causes of death in infancy. We still saw an amazing number of patients with this problem, but if we had at least four hours to work on them, we felt that we should be able to save them.

In the contagious disease unit, we saw a lot of patients with diseases that one just does not see anymore. Things like poliomyelitis, shigella dysentery, typhoid fever, tubercular meningitis, etc. We became very proficient in treating these children and very seldom lost a patient. Tubercular meningitis was known as the three-week disease because that is how long the patient usually lived. With treatment early in the disease, three weeks was how long they would stay in a coma, and then they would suddenly wake up. It was always a joyful moment when this happened. Shameful as it sounds, we saw an awful lot of diseases that killed children but were entirely preventable. This included such things as tetanus, diphtheria, whooping cough in young infants, and meningitis. This was mainly due to poor public health and the failure to institute an active immunization program.

Before telling any more war stories, I should explain terminology that doctors tend to toss around without ever explaining. Anytime that a word is used with "-itis" on the end, it means that there is inflammation of whatever precedes the "-itis." For instance, appendicitis means inflammation of the appendix from whatever cause. One needs to be somewhat familiar with the Latin roots of anatomical terms such as *myo,* which means muscle, and *car* which means heart. Put them all together, and one has myocarditis which means inflammation of the muscles of the heart. Likewise, pericarditis means inflammation of the tissues surrounding the heart. Another term that we doctors like to throw around is petechia. This is a small area of bleeding into the skin, eye, etc., which makes a spot that looks like a purple freckle. It means that blood has literally seeped through the walls of the peripheral capillaries for whatever reason.

That summer, we had sixty cases of diphtheria admitted to the isolation ward. Now this is an entirely preventable disease, and this demonstrates how inept the immunization was at that time. Diphtheria is treated with antiserum IV, huge doses of penicillin, and very close observation. The principle causes of death in diphtheria are usually one of two things: The first is blockage of the main airway by the thick, tenacious, foul-smelling membrane that forms in the mouth and throat to the point of completely blocking the trachea. The odor of diphtheria is very foul and very distinctive to diphtheria. The old story of walking into a room with diphtheria present and being able to make a diagnosis is true. The other thing that is pathognomonic of the membrane of diphtheria is the tenacity with which it clings to the tissue of the pharynx, so that it bleeds when one pulls it away. Most patients require a tracheotomy to assure a patent airway.

The other common cause of fatality is the endotoxin from the diphtheria bacteria that is infused into the body. This causes a myocarditis that essentially cannot be treated very often, either medically or surgically. Giving heart stimulants is like whipping a dead horse; it does no good. We had a small boy of about two years of age admitted with diphtheria, and subsequently, he developed myocarditis. He was nursed along and clinically recovered from his myocarditis, and after eighteen months of hospitalization, everyone thought he was all right to be discharged. In the interim between his admission and discharge, he had become the ward pet. In short, the staff had spoiled him rotten because he was a lively and thoroughly delightful child. He was released and was walking down the hospital steps when he dropped dead. Besides the overwhelming and immediate grief, a great feeling of inadequacy has always pervaded my memories of that moment.

In another example, a girl of about four years of age was brought into the emergency room with a history of collapsing in a coma; this happened while she was talking on the phone at home about thirty minutes before admission. A rapid evaluation showed the child was comatose, had petechiae scattered over her entire body, and was in shock. A presumptive diagnosis of meningococcemia was made, and after telling the mother what the diagnosis was, she was told to admit her and come straight to the isolation unit on the twelfth floor. Dr. James Coker, the pediatric resident, and I literally went running down the hall pushing a gurney with the child aboard and headed for the elevator; we rushed her to the ward and started treatment.

This disease is extremely contagious and is caused by an infection of the bloodstream and meninges of the central nervous system. This is the disease for which everyone who goes to college is reminded to get a booster shot because of the high incidence of meningitis with this germ in college-aged people. This is one of those diseases from which you either die quickly or you recover rapidly with proper therapy. In this case the child died within minutes after being admitted, and by the time the mother arrived, the child was dead. When we told her, she fell face down on the floor and began screaming and wailing while beating her fists on the floor. She was screaming, "Lordy Jesus, help me Jesus!" and "Oh, Lord!" This went on for at least ten minutes when she suddenly sat straight up, looked at us completely dry-eyed, and said, "Can I get my deposit back?"

I spent one month in the Crippled Children's Hospital, which was across the street from the front of University Hospital. This hospital was devoted to the care of children with chronic illnesses causing debilitation. The hospital was constructed so that each floor was narrower in width than the floor below. This left space for an outdoor terrace on each floor, so patients were able to be placed in the sunlight in their wheelchairs. The principal purpose of the hospital was to care for children who had recovered from poliomyelitis, but who suffered the crippling effects of spinal cord damage.

However, other patients were constantly being referred for crippling diseases that had not been diagnosed. These were always rare things that sort of came out of left field, and I really had fun working with these patients. We saw a great deal of rickets as a result of vitamin D deficiency, as well as the pseudoparalysis of scurvy, which caused the babies to not move their legs because of the extreme pain caused by attempted movement. They always would lie flat on their backs with their legs in the frog position. With a look of extreme anxiety on their faces, they would scream in pain if moved. One dose of vitamin C, and the next morning all of their pain was gone. Their pathological findings such as hemorrhages under the outer lining of the bones were still present, but the pain was gone.

The quantity of interesting patients was so large, and the likelihood of seeing another such patient anytime soon was so slight, we began to have weekly conferences to show it all off. This would serve me well later on in life, when I would be presented with some weird patient very similar to one that I had previously seen at Crippled Children's. Everyone would be gratifyingly impressed that I knew what ailed the patient.

During a student's tenure at the University Hospital, it was inevitable that a great deal of time would be spent going to see patients in the emergency room. As previously stated, it was affectionately known as the "hole." Everyone spent time down there helping to sew up all the wounded. At this time in history, Birmingham was a steel town. Essentially all of its economy was built around the steel mills. Birmingham was the only place in the world where all three things needed for the manufacture of steel were located in one spot. Iron ore, limestone, and coal were all mined within the environs of Birmingham. Now the iron ore is no longer mined and coal mines have pretty much petered out. The blast furnaces that previously turned the skies red when they were opened are now museums.

However, in those days the steel industry was by far the largest employer in Jefferson County. They paid their employees every Friday afternoon, and by dark most of them would be roaring drunk on rot-gut whiskey or a seemingly cheap brand of wine named Red Dagger. Apparently this wine had an alcohol content that pushed the upper limits of legality. After all, someone who drinks enough wine with an alcohol content that measures thirty proof will soon reach the same amount of alcohol as someone drinking forty proof whiskey. Another favorite was taking the material burned in a chafing dish or heat containers and straining it through a loaf of white bread. This would assure a state of stupor that would last for hours. If a person consumed it without the bread straining, they would be brought into the emergency room in a deep coma and found to have a blood sugar level of 0 percent. The street name for this was "Joe Louis," the heavyweight champion of the world.

After everyone reached his or her alcohol saturation point fights would inevitably break out. The favorite weapons were switchblades or straight razors. Combatants would fight until someone drew blood. Then everyone would pile into a car, and they would bring the victim to the “hole.” The “hole” was located in the north end of the condemned Hillman Hospital on the first floor. There was a small, uncovered, ambulance entrance that curved in to allow the ambulance or other vehicle to park parallel to the doors of the hospital. Brick restraining walls were constructed along the entry and exit ramps, and these served as seated waiting areas for friends and family of the combatants whenever the weather permitted. On weekend nights there was an aura of a large street party, as large groups of people would congregate. This brought on the entrepreneurs, and vendors would be selling popcorn, soft drinks, hot dogs, hamburgers, and so forth. A real party atmosphere was always evident.

The knifing party would arrive during this entire hubbub. The victim would be unloaded, go through triage, and placed somewhere until he or she could be cared not only for in order of arrival and the severity of their wounds. Medical students and house staff would go down to help with the multitudes and to become more proficient in their suturing skills. On weekends, the police had one officer assigned to work in the emergency room at night in case of belligerent behavior by a patient. After working in such circumstances for many years now, I’ve decided that there are two kinds of drunks. There are those that are happy and everybody’s friend, and those who are belligerent. A lot of times while the medical team was working on a belligerent one, the patient would get up and want to fight some more. The police officer would be called in. He would enter the room, draw his billy club and whack the guy over the head. We would put him back down on the table, restrain him, and usually he would now have a new wound requiring suturing on his head. When the victims were asked who cut them, they would answer, “My friend ‘stobbed’ me.”

I was working on a guy one night whose wife had hit him in the head with an axe during a minor marital spat. She had laid open his scalp from the forehead to the back. The skin had peeled back from the laceration and bare skull was showing for all to see. Fortunately, the axe hadn’t cracked his thick skull, and as I deadened and cleaned the wound I began to make conversation. “How did you get this cut?” I asked him.

He replied, "My wife hit me with an ax."

I said, "What? Your wife hit you with an ax?"

He looked at me as if I were completely stupid and said, "Lawdy, Doc, ain't you and your wife never had no disagreements?"

The house staff quarters were located on the seventeenth floor of the Jefferson building, which was the top floor of the center tower. To get to the emergency room one had to take the elevator down to the sixth floor, walk across a corridor to the Hillman building, catch another elevator to the bottom floor, and then walk about three-quarters of the width of the hospital to the emergency room. When one got called at two or three o'clock in the morning to come see a child, one usually tried to make that trek without completely waking up along the way. I recall making this trip on a very early morning, walking into the examining room, and saying to the very young mother, "Well Mother, what is wrong with your baby?"

She looked at me and said, "Doctor, when he cries, his navel sticks out."

Eventually I was transferred back to Children's Hospital for another rotation. It was during this rotation that I became acquainted with one of the most remarkable individuals that I have ever known. Dr. John Simpson was a very small man physically, probably not weighing more than one hundred ten pounds, which covered a frame probably five-foot, eight-inches in height. He almost always had a shy grin on his face, which could hardly be seen because of the enormous mustache that covered his upper lip. His eyes would crinkle when he smiled, and they were covered by steel-rimmed round lenses of the type worn by Harry Potter in his films. Dr. Simpson had a solo private practice which earned him enough to pursue his dedicated calling. He devoted himself to the care of patients with hydrocephalus and children with cerebral palsy.

At that time, there were no treatments available for these children. He founded a home for these children in Birmingham where they were cared for and nursed tenderly, for there was nothing else that could be done. Hydrocephalus is caused by a blockage of the flow of cerebrospinal fluid through the central nervous system. This is usually caused by a blockage of one draining duct or another, and just like your plumbing at home, the fluid begins to back up. The problem is that there is no place for the fluid to overflow, as it does with your plumbing, and this results in an enlargement of the fluid-containing areas of the brain. Due to the pressure over time the head would grow to enormous size and become very heavy; and because of the child's inability to move his head, there was a great tendency for skin breakdown and pressure sores to develop, despite the best efforts of a dedicated nursing staff.

When this did occur, the parents would have to pick up the child in their car and transport the infant to the hospital for more definitive care. They would arrive and bring their child in for admission, usually with the mother carrying the tiny body of the child and the father carrying the huge, heavy head. Sometimes they would bring the child in a wheelbarrow because the head was just too heavy for them to carry. The child would be admitted to the isolation unit, where they would be in a private room and be free from curiosity seekers. Sometimes, before the pressure sores could be adequately treated, they would erode into the cranial cavity through the gaps between the vastly separated skull bones. Cerebrospinal fluid would flow from the skull and literally flood the room. We would be paddling around in it while caring for the child. The skull would collapse to what should be the proper size for this size infant and the child would go right on living.

Nowadays, a shunt is placed in the brain to circumvent the blockage, and the child can expect a normal if slow development. Dr. John devoted his life to caring for these children, and to providing all the possible benefits of rehabilitation for cerebral palsy patients. Later, Dr. John and I wrote to all the various places which offered high-cost rehabilitation programs that claimed to help cerebral palsy patients reach their utmost potential. Not a one would give their permission for us to use their techniques, nor would they give us the protocol for performing their techniques in a program intended to compare theirs, along with other intense physical and costly programs, with simple physical therapy aimed at keeping the joints loose and range of motion as free as possible. Later, in retrospective studies, it was shown that they all reached their potential with no advantage to the costly programs, other than they reached their potential just a little sooner. Dr. John, unlike me, was not disheartened by this. He had been disappointed too many times to let one little setback affect his humor.

A while later I got a lesson in optimism from Dr. John. I came into the pediatric offices one morning to find Dr. John busily writing away on some type of document, and I said, "What are you working on, Dr. John?"

He answered, "I'm making myself a ten-year plan." He was in his middle-to-late eighties at the time, and he was dead serious.

Several years later, when I was at the University of Arkansas Medical Center in the vice president's office, I walked into my office one day and seated there in my waiting room was a little man with a shy grin on his face beneath a big bushy mustache. I guess I was more than a little homesick and feeling more than a little sorry for myself, because I have never been so glad to see anyone in my life. He said he had been missing me, and he just thought he would drive up to see me. Nothing important was going on, just dropped in to see a friend. It was quite an emotional moment for me, I'll tell you.

I continued my rotation at Children's with nothing unusual happening until we admitted a little boy with an incurable disease. After consulting with many people, we determined there just wasn't anything that we could do to help this young fellow. Suddenly, someone was telling me that I needed to tell the mother. I had never done this before. Dewey, who had done this many times in his lifetime, told me that I just needed to explain the situation to her and what the outcome was going to be. I can close my eyes and see her clearly, just as she was that day. She was a young blond girl of about twenty years in a cheap, very plain dress with stark fear etched on her face. I started out all right while I was explaining about the child's condition, but then I came to the part where I had to give her a prognosis. Then I began to hem and haw, beat around the bush, and do anything that postponed the inevitable. I could clearly see that I was keeping her in agony while I kept skirting around the truth. Finally, she asked me a direct question: "Is my son going to live?"

I couldn't run away from that, and I answered in a voice so low that even I had trouble hearing it; "No." I finally got it out. As mothers seem prone to do in these moments, she turned her back to me, put her hands to her mouth, and cried silently. I was keenly aware that I had made the horrible news worse by my actions, and I vowed to never put anyone through that ordeal again. Since that time, I have had to impart that message again and again. I would like to tell you that it gets easier with time and repetitions, but it doesn't. Now I start off telling the parents that I have some very grave news for them, and then tell them the awful prognosis. I have been criticized by family onlookers for being so brief, but you can believe me, I know drawing it out does not make it better.

Throughout my internship, I kept running into three fellows

from the senior class, Charlie Alford, Bill Benton, and Hugh Dillon. Hugh was destined to be my best friend, and all three of them and I had the destiny of having our futures closely entwined. I had decided to stay put for my residency, and I encouraged the three of them to take a straight pediatric internship, which they did. None of us could envision what our futures held.

My first year of pediatric residency started out with my being very comfortable about the whole situation. I had gotten a raise to one-hundred and twenty-five dollars a month, and my confidence in my ability to handle any situation presented to me in the pediatric field was never higher. In fact, this time in my life portrays my utmost level of confidence. Since that moment, my confidence in my ability has steadily eroded. It is what I like to call the arrogance of ignorance. One doesn't know enough to know how little one knows. You see this often in people with surgical personalities. The year went very smoothly, with the three straight interns superbly holding up their end of the labor.

Hugh Dillon and I began to work together a lot, merely due to the luck of the draw in the working schedule. Hugh was a native of Auburn, Alabama. His father, who had died early in Hugh's life, had been on the faculty of the veterinary school. One will never meet a bigger Auburn fan than he was. His mother ran a boarding house for students in their family home, and Hugh had friends at every level of academic prowess, due to knowing them when they slept and ate in his home. Hugh was a very outgoing person and knew an extraordinary number of people. I don't think there was ever a time when we walked into a restaurant that as we were being seated he would not say, "Excuse me a minute; I want to speak to these people over there."

His father-in-law owned a cattle farm outside Childersburg, Alabama, which had large and small ponds that were stocked with bass and bream, but their real purpose was supposedly for irrigation of the pasture grass and the corn crop if needed. I can assure you they were used for fishing a lot more than they were supposed to be. The land also had quail and the migration of doves, and his father-in-law just happened to have an Irish setter quail dog. Hugh had been doing all of these things since growing up in Auburn, and he showed me the ropes. I had never bird-hunted before and had only squirrel-hunted with a .22 rifle.

Through our years together, he made me into a fair bird-shooter and fly-fisher. We were lucky in another way also. One of the boys that boarded with his mother was "Shug" Jordan, who became head coach at Auburn about the time Hugh and I started to become friends. In addition, an assistant line coach's wife was close friends with Hugh's wife, Lil. That gave us two entrees into football tickets. Hugh would hand me a sideline pass, which we would attach to our coats, and we watched many wonderful ball games from the sidelines. Hugh and I had many wonderful times together in those days. He has been dead several years now, and I miss him terribly. You will hear many tales about Hugh in this tome of recollections. We stuck together through thick and thin.

Sometime in these residency years, Mac Bargeron joined the faculty. Mac finished his training at Columbia and came down to Birmingham to start a pediatric cardiology program. He studied under Dr. Richmond Bing, an internist, and one of the pioneers in cardiac catheterization. Dr. Bing was on the medical faculty at Alabama, and he set up one of the first catheterization clinics in the South. Mac took over the pediatric program, and it was one of my favorite and most productive rotations.

When I finished my first year residency, I suddenly started to hear from my draft board. They allowed two years of postgraduate study and then the student was expected to apply for a commission in the service of his choice. I talked to several people, and they all assured me that the Air Force was the best service for physicians. I knew I didn't want to go into the Navy as I get seasick in a bathtub. So I applied to the Air Force and so notified the Draft Board. A few weeks went by and I got a reply from the Air Force. They stated that they had all the doctors they needed at the present time, but to apply later when they were sure there would be openings. I innocently wrote the Draft Board and reported what the Air Force had told me. I informed them that I would reapply after waiting a little while.

Well, I got back this snotty letter from the Draft Board stating that if I didn't apply to another branch of the armed services soon, I would be inducted as a buck private in the rear ranks. After a few seconds, I got the message and reluctantly applied for a commission in the Army. After a while, I got all the forms from the Army. While looking at the multiple pages, I got an inspiration: Why don't I just "forget" to fill out one of the many pages and send it in blank, with all the remaining forms filled in correctly. I mailed them off, and in about three months I got a reply saying that I had omitted filling out one page, and would I fill it in and mail it back. This I did, but I "forgot" to sign them, and then I dutifully mailed them. After a while, I got the expected reply, and I sent it back one more time with something else wrong. By this time I figured I had run this about as long as I could. I reapplied to the Air Force, and this time they had openings. I applied, got my forms, filled them out (correctly this time), and was soon accepted. Hugh swore me in, as he was a reserve officer, and now I had become a captain in the military service of our country.

I received another set of forms to fill out, and they told me how to list my preferences for an Air Force base. I wrote down all the exotic places that were listed, and when I got my orders I was assigned to Barksdale AFB in Shreveport, Louisiana. I never thought of it before, but perhaps they corresponded with the Army about me. I'm sure that they thought I was the dumbest doctor they had ever had apply.

In January, 1954, I left Birmingham and began my two years of active military service.

Unknown to me at the time, the federal government was beginning to involve itself in the furthering of medical research by funding the National Institutes of Health in Bethesda, Maryland. This has been proven to be a wonderful investment, with its programs being directed by physicians and other scientists. There are brilliant investigators working in the various institutes with great accomplishments in a myriad of scientific endeavor. In addition, individual research grants were awarded to individual investigators in various universities and institutes. This was accomplished by doing some prior experimental work on a problem that one had become involved in and had some positive findings that needed further work.

One would apply for a research grant by detailing the question to be answered, what work and the findings of that work one had already done, details of the method of experimentation that one intended to pursue, and finally, a proposed budget for the money requested. A panel of one's peers is formed to evaluate the proposal along with the ability of thc applicant to carry the project. The panel consists of scientific leaders in the field in which this proposed experimental project falls. After discussing the project, the proposed methodology projected to be used by the applicant, and the investigator's scientific ability to carry this out, the application is then awarded or disapproved by the panel. At this point the only politics in the procedure takes place. The information is forwarded to the senior senator from the applicant's state and he or she notifies the press, the university, and the applicant. I don't know if this has changed any, though I would suspect that politics has found a way to destroy the pristine nature of it.

Also, block grants were made available for universities where several investigators were working on the same project, and one block grant to the school would cover the needs of them all.

Another facet of federal involvement was the passage of the Hill-Burton Act for the construction of hospitals that were needed in individual states. In each state, there was a panel appointed from the state medical association to determine need, type of facility, and just the feasibility of a proposed hospital. The principal aim of the legislation was to provide hospitals for rural areas and specialty hospitals for possible referrals. Since Senator Hill was Alabama's senior senator, the state probably got more than its share of the money. The interest in medicine, which was shown by Senator Hill, was easily understood. His father was a surgeon who trained under Lister, the father of antiseptic surgery. There was no surprise when he named Senator Hill after Lister. His father was also the first physician to suture a beating heart. One of his patients was stabbed, which created a small hole in the ventricle of his heart. He opened the man's chest and pericardium and closed the hole with one suture. He then closed the pericardium and chest wall, and the fellow lived to fight again.

Chapter 7

Military Career — A Good Soldier, I Was Not

I had to drive down to Gunter Air Force Base in Montgomery, Alabama for my induction. I was housed in the BOQ (bachelors officers' quarters), ate in the mess hall, and attended classes telling us how to behave as officers. We received a good bit of money for housing, uniforms, etc., and I felt like I was really rich with all that cash in my pockets for a change. I was still being thrifty, however. In the Air Force, airmen only had to wear a dress uniform in the winter months. At some time, the powers that be would send down a directive telling everyone that it was time to switch to summer uniforms or vice versa. With the summer uniform, one had only to wear khaki pants and short-sleeved shirts open at the collar. Dress uniforms were required only at formal affairs. I wasn't planning on going to any formal affairs, so I didn't buy one. I figured I saved myself a hundred and fifty dollars to apply to better things.

After two weeks, I had to drive over to Barksdale and report for duty. I checked into the BOQ and drove over to the hospital. The first day was taken up with picture taking, meeting people, and being shown around by the guy that I was replacing. He left the next day, and I was in charge of the pediatric department which included me, me, and only me. I thought that I would make fast rounds, check the nursery, and then go over to housing to get us an apartment on base. The officer's quarters were two-story duplexes, unless one considered the huge homes in the old part of the base where the senior officers lived.

While making nursery rounds I noticed that a slightly premature baby looked a little yellow, especially for one less than twenty-four-hours old. We checked his blood and determined that he had hemolytic anemia of the newborn and was going to need an exchange transfusion. I had done several of these procedures, since we did the first one that was ever done in Alabama. I went out to talk with the father, a master sergeant, and the mother. I explained the situation and told them that even though the child was a little premature, I didn't expect any difficulty. We proceeded with the transfusion, which ordinarily lasts about an hour, and finished right on time. The baby did stop breathing a couple of times but was easily started back. We finished, and I went out and told the parents everything was fine, and we probably would not have any more trouble (and we didn't).

I was then free to go over to housing and get Nancy and me a place to live. I found the right building and walked in. There, sitting behind the counter was a master sergeant whom I recognized as the father of the baby who had just had the exchange transfusion. He said, "Don't worry, Doc. I'll get you a good place to live."

About an hour later he called me at the hospital and shouted, "Doc, I got you a great place. It's right next door to the General." He had gotten me one of those huge houses next door to the base commander. I told him that I didn't have enough furniture to fill up the living room. I really appreciated his efforts, but I really just needed a two-bedroom apartment in Wherry housing. He really didn't understand it, but he found me what I asked for.

We moved into our new digs, and gradually we got our feet on the ground. We found the Base Exchange (BX) and the commissary, which was kind of like a present-day Sam's, Wal-Mart's big wholesale stores. The hospital contained a general pediatric ward for all ages and two private rooms for contagious cases. There was a general nursery and a very small premature nursery containing two or three isolette incubators.

The pediatric clinic was in a clapboard building attached to the hospital. This was a standard government building that was long and relatively narrow, with a fairly wide hall down the center. There was a waiting area at the far end of the building, and there were examining rooms on each side of the hall. The emergency room was strategically located in the other end of the building where it was closest to the hospital. There was no drive-in area for an ambulance to get close to the only door. I only saw the base ambulance bring in a patient on two separate occasions, and each time the corpsmen just carried the litter up the short steps into the emergency. One of these occasions was a young airman who dropped dead while playing basketball, and we never took him out of the center hall. I pronounced him dead in the hall and they turned around and took him to the morgue.

We had to eat hospital food when we were on duty. It wasn't too bad, actually. Each day, one of the staff physicians was Medical Officer of the Day (MOD), and we were on duty for thirty-six hours straight. We had a MOD room in the hospital where the corpsmen or nurses could get the physician if needed. There was no phone in the room for some reason, and if you were needed, a nurse or corpsman would wake you up by gently shaking your shoulder. Something like officer's privilege or something, I guess.

The MOD saw everyone who came in, regardless of the nature of the problem. Since I had not taken care of any adults since medical school it was a little awkward initially, but it all came back rather rapidly. I could call for help from one of the specialties if the situation so dictated. When I was off, I rarely got called except when the psychiatrist was MOD. He was totally insecure when it came to medical problems, especially when they were in children.

He was really an interesting person. He was born and raised in Brooklyn, New York, and had never been out of Brooklyn in all of his life. He had never driven a car, but when he was assigned his duty station at Barksdale, he bought himself a new car, learned to drive it, and drove himself and his family all the way to northwestern Louisiana. He marveled at all the vacant space that existed between home and Barksdale. He said, "Everyone talks about shortage of space for the future generations. Why, there is just an immense amount of space out there to put people." It was nothing like Brooklyn.

I found that the families of airmen were usually woefully lacking in getting the proper immunizations for their children. The Air Force furnished free day care for the dependent children, both during the day or at night. I thought, well, this offers us an opportunity to insure proper immunizations of the children. With all my executive power as head of the pediatric services on base, I issued an executive order that no child could use the nursery or day care services unless they were up to date on their immunizations or were in the process of receiving their immunizations. Problem solved.

It was only then I learned that there were no well-baby services offered on the base. What I had envisioned as a good thing turned into just as big a problem as the one I thought I was solving. Well, I wasn't going to rescind my previous executive order. I would lose face. There was only one way to solve this: we would establish well-baby services. With more than a little help from a few master sergeants, I got the space (remember my sergeant over at housing) which was far enough away from the hospital environment with all of its germs, equipment, staff, and records. We were in business. I wrote down the immunization schedule and posted it, and once again the problem was solved.

That led to my first congressional investigation (I wasn't really too good a soldier). In the Air Force if *anyone* was dissatisfied about something that was happening, he could complain to his congressman. To show that he was definitely interested in any problem that they might have, the congressperson would instigate an investigation. This involved writing your commanding officer and telling him to look into the problem and solve it. It seems that the recommendations of the Academy of Pediatrics were different from the Air Force immunization schedule. The colonel called me in and told me that I could use the recommendations of the Academy if I wanted to, but just don't write it down. I suppose that some person familiar with our procedures in the well-baby clinic didn't like our not going by Air Force immunization rules. There always seems to be one of those types who thinks, "We have never done it like that before." How many times I have heard that in my life? I took down all the signs, we continued as we were doing, and the problem was really solved this time.

Shortly after getting to Barksdale we learned that Nancy was pregnant with our first son, Paul Crawford. The Paul is from me, and the Crawford is from Nancy's maternal family. The obstetrician on the base was Nick Parapid, a major in the regular Air Force. He was a good doctor, but he said that Nancy would do better to go to private obstetricians in town. She went to one that was recommended and was pleased as could be. The obstetrician was one of those fairly good-looking men who called his patients, "darling," and patted their hands. The pediatrician was the fellow in town who was my consultant for pediatric problems I might have on the base. The pregnancy and delivery went smoothly. Nancy didn't even know that she had delivered when she awoke the next morning. The only thing that bothered me was that Paul looked an awful like my father-in-law. However, he grew out of it. Later on, I told my father-in-law how relieved I was. He and I were great buddies.

As anyone who has had a child will tell you, your life is never the same after a child arrives. Paul was a very good baby. He never had colic, and if he was fretful and wouldn't go to sleep, we would put him in his little bed in the car and he would be asleep before we would get around the block.

My life on the base was generally unexciting. We got in a new man without a specialty ranking and the colonel asked him if he would like to go on the pediatric service. This was a fellow from Holland, Michigan. He had no predilection for pediatrics, but it just seemed to him to be an easy service, I think. The service had gotten a lot busier by then. People had started to take their children to the base for care rather than the private sector. You know, build a better mousetrap and the world will beat a path to your door. Jim took to pediatrics like a duck to water. He enjoyed it immensely, and after the Air Force he served his pediatrics residency at the University of Michigan. He settled in Holland to practice and built a very successful practice. Ultimately, his oldest son went into pediatrics, and the latest I heard his grandson was also a pediatrician. They all practice together where Jim started his practice. Later in my life, when Ray Peterson and I were doing our research on lymphatic leukemia, Jim asked me to come up to Michigan to give a talk to the pediatric society down at Ann Arbor, Michigan. I stayed with them in Holland and we had a very nice time recalling old experiences. I haven't seen or heard from him since.

During the first year at Barksdale, we moved off the base to a small house in Bossier City, Louisiana. The noise of bombers taking off and landing was very irritating to Nancy. The house was only a hop, skip, and jump from the base's east gate, but it was fairly well removed from the flight line. Our landlord was the obstetrician from the base. He owned our house and the one he lived in next door. We were always doing projects together, mainly in our carport. We built a small boat from some plans that he had, again using our carport. As I remember, it was about seven-feet long and had a wooden covering over the bow, but it was wide enough to be stable in the water.

We gave it the ultimate test after Nick had gone solo on the water. We took it out to Lake Bistenau outside Shreveport. This was one of the lakes in Louisiana that are part of one huge swamp system. It was a huge lake with extremely few areas of open water. The remainder was cypress swamp water with huge cypress trees every few feet, and it was a bass fisherman's dream. When we both got in that little boat, it reminded me of the nursery rhyme about three men in a tub. I must admit that it handled the water extremely well, and we fished for bass with yellow sally lures. I hate to mention it, but I skunked him. I had five big, big bass, and he had one little scrawny one. Funny, but I don't remember him asking me to go with him anymore.

Barksdale was a SAC (Strategic Air Command) base under the command of the infamous General Curtis LeMay. He was the commander in the Pacific Theater who ordered the firebombing of Tokyo and literally burned most of it to the ground. Later he would give the final orders to drop the A-Bombs on Japan. With him in command, SAC was a spit and polish outfit. It was the height of the Cold War, and planes were kept in ready condition to fly at a moment's notice.

Inside Barksdale AFB was another base named Bossier Base. This was surrounded by three ten-foot fences topped with rolls of razor wire. The middle fence was electrified with high-voltage electricity. One night when I was MOD, an airman, who was drunk out of his mind, climbed the outer fence and, after cutting his skin to ribbons climbing over the razor wire, was found standing between the outer fence and the middle fence. The guards yelled at him to stand still and definitely not to touch the middle fence before they could get the electricity turned off. He stood up, laughed, and staggered back into the electrified fence. They brought his body into the emergency room, but it was just a smoldering mass of charcoal.

Bossier Base was also patrolled by German shepherd guard dogs. Each dog had one handler, and each dog would not let anyone but that individual handle him. The MPs were constantly bringing in their comrades who had fallen and were subsequently dragged by their dogs. They would be scratched and gouged all over from the dragging. This was the area in which the atom bombs were stored.

When I first arrived, B-47s were being flown by the flight crews. They had a crew of three: the pilot, the co-pilot, and a navigator operating the aircraft. Whenever some suspicious blip was seen on the radar stations located across the northern regions of America, these and other planes from SAC stations all over the world would take off with a designated bombing target and an atomic bomb in the belly of the plane. Canadian bush pilots must have cost the United States millions of dollars during the years of the Cold War, because every time one would take off from some forlorn Canadian arctic lake all the bombers in SAC would take off.

Now, when these planes took off a thing called a general alert was called. Everyone had a specific duty to perform to get those planes into the air and on their way. For doctors, it meant getting to the base, going on the flight line, and doing physical exams on any flying personnel who might be ailing. If someone tried to fly with a good deal of nasal congestion, it could lead to ruptured eardrums if there was a rapid descent and change in the air pressure. When they called an alert I didn't have any specific duties, the cause of which is a long story. In SAC, planes were constantly flying to far-off bases, and the physicians could catch a flight on a tanker and spend days in some foreign land. When the tanker returned to home base, they came back. too. Everyone was eligible to do this but me—the reason being that I was the only pediatrician on the base, and the colonel wouldn't let me be away that long. In retaliation, I never got a flight line pass, and therefore I couldn't go on the flight line to examine personnel. I spent two years of active duty in the Air Force and never set foot in a plane. It was kind of a Russian standoff with neither side bending.

One day, one of the people who did get to make one of those excursions came up to me and said, "I met a fellow over in North Africa who says that he knows you, and he sends his regards. His name is George Bilsten." George was one of those true characters to whom things were always happening. His family were German Jews who escaped Germany barely in time to miss the concentration camps. He graduated from medical school at the University of Washington, and he decided to come to the University of Alabama for his postgraduate training.

While driving from Washington to Alabama, he was going through one of the national parks out West spotted a coyote along the roadside. He stopped his car, got out to take a picture, and the coyote ran over and bit him. He took his picture and showed it to us while on pediatrics, but he had to take rabies shots since there was no way to tell whether the coyote was rabid or not. When he rotated onto the pediatric service, part of the time was spent on the infectious disease unit. It was during a time when we were having a small epidemic of whooping cough. George caught it. There is an old saying about whooping cough: it is three weeks coming, three weeks here and three weeks leaving.

When George got over that, he started a neurology residency. When electroencephalograms (EEG) are done, the neurology residents have to read them and get a report to the referring physician quickly. One day, the head of neurology called George and said, "Dr. Bilsten, your EEG box is overflowing with unread EEGs. What do you think we ought to do?"

George replied earnestly, "Dr. Little, I suggest that you get a bigger box."

The Colonel and I really got along very well. I kept the pediatric service running smoothly, and no one was worried about his children getting the proper care. This saved him a lot of personnel headaches. We did have a tragic thing happen while I was stationed at Barksdale. One of the colonel's two children was struck and run over by the base fire truck. It was just one of those tragic accidents that occur with small children. Well, they had the funeral on the base and it was a formal affair, so I had to go down and buy that formal dress uniform. It truly was the only time that I wore it.

As the time of my tour of active duty grew shorter, I had to start thinking about what I was going to do when I got out. I still had my dream of practicing pediatrics in a small town. In the interim, Hugh Dillon had gone to the University of Minnesota to finish his pediatric training. He kept writing and calling me, telling me how great the training was. He knew of my interest in hematology, and he had spoken to the pediatric hematologist-oncologist about a possible fellowship for me. He also kept urging me to think about it. I wasn't too attracted to that idea, however, and I started looking at places I might practice. I looked into Hattiesburg, Mississippi, and Fairhope, Alabama, along with several others, and I couldn't find any other place that offered any encouragement. So after talking about it, Nancy, Paul, and I headed out to the frozen region of the University of Minnesota. We stopped along the way in the outskirts of St. Louis, Missouri, and bought Nancy and Paul the proper overshoes for walking in snow. They didn't have such things in Louisiana or Alabama.

All in all, my time spent on active duty was not bad. I didn't particularly like the restriction of travel without permission, but I got used to it. I would eventually spend four more years in the Inactive Reserves before receiving my honorable discharge. While in Minnesota and later in Alabama, I kept getting letters telling me that if I didn't switch from Inactive Reserves to Active Reserves, my chances for promotion were essentially nil. Later, when I was attending a Society for Pediatric Research meeting in Seattle, Washington, I was explaining this to Heinz Eichenwald, who was then chairman of the Department of Pediatrics at Southwestern School of Medicine in Dallas, Texas. He said, "Oh, don't worry about that. I get those letters all the time from the Public Health Service. I expect to wake up any day and find out that I have been made surgeon general." I held the rank of lieutenant colonel when I got my discharge papers.

When I left Barksdale, I got a citation for my good work on base. I suppose that I did leave the quality of pediatric care a little better than I found it. That is what I was hoping would be the story of my life as I proceeded through my pediatric career. At that moment, though, I was entering a world of pediatrics I had never even thought about entering and really knew very little about.

Chapter 8

Postdoctoral Fellowship — The Learning of Medicine as a Profession not a Trade

Dr. Bill Krivit, my new mentor, had found us a place to rent in St. Louis Park, Minnesota. The house belonged to the mother of Bill's lab technician. We got it at a very reasonable rate, and it afforded us all the room that we needed. The place had a basement underneath the entire house, which cut down on heating costs. We had our hide-a-bed couch put down there, and any guests who visited us were housed down there. The basement also held a gas-fired, hot-air furnace which kept us toasty warm even when sub-zero temperatures prevailed for days on end. Upstairs there were four rooms, all equal in size. These were the living room, the kitchen with a small dining area, two bedrooms, and a tiny bath. It didn't seem so small when we moved in, but when confined for days on end because of the cold, it became very conducive to cabin fever. Since we lived so far from the university, I had to drive the car to work every weekday, and this left Nancy no escape. We arrived in the middle of January, and that meant it would be another five months before the spring thaw and people started peeking out from their homes.

When we arrived, it was what they call up there a spring day. The high for the day was thirty-two degrees, and I thought that this wasn't going to be so bad. The movers were two huge Swedes who pretty much carried everything solo, with only one of them carrying a large piece of furniture. When it came time to take the refrigerator into the house, I thought that surely they would use a freight dolly to roll it in. No way. One of the guys walked up to it, threw a sling around it, backed up to the refrigerator and heaved the piece on his back, walked into the kitchen where he gently set it down. I made a mental note to stay on the good side of them.

The next morning when we awoke, it was twenty degrees below zero. I went out to the car, and when I turned the ignition key the engine kind of groaned and managed about two revolutions. Amazingly, the engine fired up and was ready to go. They put some sort of additive in every brand of gasoline, so if the driver could coax one spark out of the engine, it would fire off. The next trouble I found was when I started to drive down the street: with every rotation of a wheel there was a bump. Finally it dawned on me that my tires had frozen, and where the tire had been sitting on the ground was frozen flat. Every time the wheel turned and it came to the flat area on all four tires, there was a more-than-slightly discernible bump. It took several blocks before the tires would round out.

I reported to work the first morning at the pediatric offices. Nancy and I had driven up and spent a few days in the fall, so I knew most of the people. I was given a desk in an office with Bill Krivit and the fellow who ran the residency program over at Minneapolis General Hospital, where the pediatrics residents regularly rotated. Bill spent a lot of time complaining about this guy hanging his suit coats so that the Hong Kong tailor label on the inside of the jacket always showed. He was a very pleasant fellow, though, and we really didn't see much of him.

I didn't know what to expect in my training agenda. In just a few days it became obvious to me that everyone in the pediatric program had several research projects. To go from a program where no one had a research project to one where everybody had one or more projects was quite a change in philosophy for me to wrap my brain around. The quality of the faculty was another thing that astounded me. Every faculty member was a renowned figure in his or her field. There was an abundance of patients from all over the world who had been referred in for diagnosis and treatment.

We weren't dealing with acute illnesses from the clinic or the emergency room. All of those were taken care of at Minneapolis General Hospital. We were dealing with children with diseases that may not even have been described yet. I slowly began to understand the concept of "experiments of nature." Children were referred to us because there was a problem with some small part of the normal physiology in that child that was not functioning as it should. This resulted in a disease process. The basic question would be, "What exactly is not working and why?" The challenge was to first discover what exactly wasn't working in a particular system in the child's body. A lot of times the answer could not be given because no one knew how that particular system worked.

The researchers would then "take the problem to the laboratory bench." They would begin a study of this particular system in humans and in the appropriate experimental animal. When they had at least a rudimentary knowledge of this particular system in the normal, they could then see what part of that system wasn't present or not functioning in the patient. In this manner, the faulty system was identified along with what parts of that particular system were determined to be missing, or not functioning, in this particular pathologic identity. A classic example from medical history is the young boy who was having repeated infections for no obvious reasons. His very astute personal physician found he did not have any demonstrable gamma globulin in his blood stream. From this initial observation the entire immune system has been virtually identified and the intricate interactions of its innumerable components described. This work was led principally by the research of Dr. Robert A. Good, the Variety Club Professor of Pediatrics, at the University of Minnesota.

This thinking was something entirely new for me. The concept of not being satisfied with just attaching a name to a patient's problem, but actually delving into and identifying the altered physiology that was the cause of the disease was an entirely new way to think and act. If psychiatrists had approached their patients' problems this way instead of rehashing theories proposed in the late 1800s, their patients would be far better off today.

I hadn't been thinking this way, so I didn't have any research thoughts in mind when I began. Bill started me off with some simple projects that needed to be done and they would keep my mind and me busy. In the meantime, he gave me a research project of my own so I would have some results to talk about. The first project took me back to the same subject that I always seemed to start new careers with–exchange transfusions. In the usual transfusion, the baby's blood was typed and cross-matched with donor blood that was preserved in an ACD solution containing an anticoagulant to keep the blood from clotting, citrate to slightly acidify the blood (which makes the red cells survive longer in storage), and dextrose to give the red cells some food on which they could survive.

For a period of time, the pediatric department at Minnesota had been using heparin as an anticoagulant. This gave the freedom from having to give periodic injections of potassium to avoid the possible stopping of the heart. I went back and reviewed all the charts of patients where heparin was used as an anticoagulant, along with those that had occurred since I arrived. We accumulated all the data, and I wrote my first published article, "The Use of Heparinized Blood in Exchange Transfusion." I was as proud as a peacock, but I will admit that I was surprised to hear from former colleagues that they too had read it and complimented me on it.

Another task was to report a child with a very rare form of childhood leukemia, called eosinophilic leukemia. I was told to do a little research on the subject, and we would submit it to a journal. Well, you know how I was taught by my parents: if you are going to do something, do it right. So, I did a survey of the world's literature on eosinophilic leukemia. There were a lot of German articles written on the subject, and essentially the only German words I knew were "*ja*" and "*nein.*" However, there was a pediatric resident who had spent two years in Germany on his missionary service in the Mormon Church. He said he didn't speak a word of German when he went over, but necessity dictated that he must learn to be fluent in both speaking and reading the language.

I would check the journals out of the library, grab my friend, go up to my desk, and make notes while he read the article to me. I had all the differential diagnoses laid out, and it turned out to be a very long article when all the microscopic pictures of the bone marrow, etc., were added in. We sent it to the *Journal of Medicine* and I thought, "No one is going to read this thing because it is too long." We had to order reprints three times because of the number of requests for them. We sent out over a thousand! You have to remember that I was new at this business. Bill Krivit explained to me that the physicians who read *The Journal of Medicine* were known for their desires for reprints. If they wanted to reread an article, they had it near at hand. I took that to mean I shouldn't let the number of requests for it to go to my head.

Soon after arriving, Nancy and I made another discovery. With another move we had another pregnancy. This time, Nancy was taken care of by a fellow in the department of obstetrics who was recommended by Bill Krivit. Bill would take care of the baby when it came. The pregnancy went along without any major problems. The only thing was, this current obstetrician was the antithesis of the fellow Nancy had in Louisiana. It was strictly all business, very professional, and absolutely not one "darling" or patted hand. Because she had such a relatively easy time with her first delivery, Nancy was instructed to come to the hospital at the first hint of labor. We left Paul with Bill and Ann Benton, who had arrived in July in order for Bill to serve his last year of a pediatric residency. That is a story for a later time.

Nancy had John without a long labor, and only had to stay in the hospital about one and a half days. John wasn't faring so well—he wouldn't take liquids, and when he did, he vomited. It became obvious that he had an intestinal obstruction, or as they say in the clinic, he had "the locked bowels." Bill got the pediatric surgeon in, and it was decided that surgery was needed. John was taken to the operating room and they found that he had a condition known as malrotation of the large bowel with a fibrous tissue going across the duodenum, partially obstructing it. This band was severed and the colon put in its proper place. He came out of surgery with no complications, but he continued to vomit and not retain adequate food.

He was delicately nursed along by the newborn nursery staff, and after two weeks he was discharged from the hospital. He had lost close to one-half of his birth weight and he looked like a drowned rat. In the meantime, Mama had swallowed her fear of flying long enough to fly to Minneapolis to help take care of John. The first thing she did after her first Minnesota breakfast was to walk up to the small corner grocery and buy some of her Louisiana-brand of coffee. She brewed herself some black coffee strong enough that she could not see the bottom of a teaspoon when it was filled with that brew. She poured herself a cup, sat back, and let out a big sigh.

John was so scrawny that his head looked too big for his body. Mama told Nancy's mom that she thought he had a deformed head. Nancy's folks didn't see him until we got to Jacksonville at Christmas. By that time we had fattened him up, and they were relieved to find him not deformed. He was about a year old before we got him to the point where his weight matched his height and age.

All of the physicians donated the time they spent taking care of a poor hematology fellow's new son, but the hospital had to be paid for the operating room, two weeks hospitalization, etc. There wasn't any way I was going to be able to pay for that on my three-hundred dollar monthly salary. Again, Bill Krivit came to my rescue, and, after the hospital gave us a discount, he managed to get the balance paid from funds of a foundation that paid hospital costs for needy children. I'll always be grateful for his help throughout that ordeal. I would never have made it without him.

My fellowship was rolling along very well. In the spring, while Nancy was still "great with child," Bill took me to the "Young Turks" spring meeting at Atlantic City, New Jersey. This was a meeting of young internists who report on new research results from their individual research programs. This was long before the gambling empire took over Atlantic City. At this time, it was an old seaside resort town where people came with their families to spend time at the seashore. Gambling was not even legal in New Jersey at that time. Because in the early spring it was too cold to attract tourists and sea bathers, conventions were sought as a continued source of revenue.

Therefore, all the restaurants, boardwalk businesses, etc., were open just as they were in the good old summertime. Everyone wanted lobster. It was relatively cheap there, so almost every evening we went to some Captain's lobster house. One night we caught a jitney bus out to one of these places. I was sitting up front directly across the center aisle from the jitney driver. He turned to me and said, "What convention is in town?" I told him that there was a scientific conference. He replied, "I wondered. All the working girls have gone out of town for the weekend." Well, so much for our image as wild, carefree scientific conventioneers.

After the convention ended, we boarded a bus to Deal, New Jersey, where Bill's family lived just across the river from New York City. His family was like a Jewish family that had been drawn from some television program. Bill's mother was intrigued with my name, Herschel. It is a Yiddish name for Harold in English. While slowly wagging her head in disbelief, she said, "Herschel . . . Bentley, yet."

They were one of the most gracious and generous families that I have ever met. Bill's dad always went fishing on certain days of the week, and this was one of those days. He just took Bill and me along. He had rented a sea-going size boat and we fished for flounder in some bay. I really never did know where we were. We caught a bunch of flounder, and Bill's dad gave them all away. He didn't want to be bothered with having to clean them. That night we drove through the tunnel into New York City. We met Bill's sister and husband, and they all showed me the sights of Manhattan. We dined in the true sense of the word at a fine restaurant, and then we all went to see a Broadway play.

That was an entirely new experience for me. We were seated in the center section about five rows back. The play was *Zelda*, starring Jason Robards, Jr., and it was a delightful experience indeed. It is a play about F. Scott Fitzgerald's wife. Incidentally, she was from Montgomery, Alabama, and led a tormented life. She died in a psychiatric hospital in Ashville, North Carolina, while an inpatient there. She had apparently fallen asleep in bed while smoking a cigarette and was severely burned and died. To this day no patient in that hospital is allowed to have matches or cigarette lighters. The next day we flew back to Minneapolis, where I had to tell Nancy all about my sojourn into New York, etc.; at the same time that she was stuck at home.

Since I still didn't have a clue about what I might want to do as a research project, I was given one. Bill, one lab tech (her mother was our landlord), and I had one laboratory bench on which to work. It was at the far end of the hall from our offices. Situated across the hall was Dr. Lewis Wannamaker's laboratory. You will hear more about him later, but he was one of the world's authorities on streptococcal infections and the organisms themselves. His two fellows worked there also: Dr. Paul Quie, a native Minnesotan whose brother became the first Republican Governor of Minnesota, and Eliyah Ayoub, a Lebanese immigrant whose family had been ousted from their family's homestead to make way for the creation of Israel. He was not anti-Jewish, but he was certainly was anti-Zionist. Paul was working on staphylococcal infections and Eliyah was working on the body's response to different types of streptococci. Paul would later be appointed to fill the Variety Club Professor of Pediatrics endowed chair when Bob Good left to become head of research at Sloan-Kettering Institute in New York. Those are two more stories that will be covered later.

Fortunately, Bill didn't come down to the laboratory very much, and this left a little more room for the rest of us. I was given the task of devising a test for measurement of the clotting factor, Factor

8, in the circulating blood. It had to be sensitive enough to detect small deviations from normal. Factor 8 Deficiency, also known as Classical Hemophilia A, is the most common type of "free bleeders." It is carried as a gene on the X chromosome, and causes all males who inherit the hemophilia X gene from their mothers to become a hemophiliac. The problem at the time was that no one had developed a way to diagnosis the carrier state. The expression of the gene could skip generations before having a hemophilic male show up. Also, if a daughter of a known carrier wanted to have children, there was no way to say "yea" or" nay" on being a carrier. Fifty percent of the daughters of a carrier theoretically will be a carrier.

I was given an end of the lab bench on which to work. Bill had to work on a very tight budget, which meant that there would be no new equipment bought for this project. Bill's lab tech did all of the lab work done on new suspected hemophiliacs, and she was extremely good at it. She was a short, dumpy girl, a little on the chubby side. Her personality was very open and friendly, and she taught me how to do all the tests. If she hadn't been around to teach me the ropes, I doubt if I would have gotten this done. To do the clotting studies, I definitely needed a water bath to maintain all the testing substances at thirty seven degrees centigrade.

Most folks would simply go down to the laboratory supply store and buy a water bath with a dial on it to set the water at the proper temperature. That was not an option for me. We scrounged around in the supply closet and found an old electric hot plate. We also found a gallon bucket that didn't leak and, since we did have a spare centigrade thermometer, we were definitely on our way.

Through trial and error, I found that the water in the bucket had to be gently circulated or there would be water strata formed with each being a different temperature. To solve this problem I found rubber and glass tubing, and by connecting it all was able to suspend the opening just above the bottom of the bucket. I then connected the tube to the compressed air jet on the lab table, and again through trial and error determined exactly how much air to pass through the tube to make the water keep a steady 37 degrees C. I carefully marked the spot on the air jet and the dial on the hot plate so I was now able to reproduce 37 degrees consistently. I suspended a wire test tube rack in the water, and I was in business.

There is a factor in red cells that when released by the breakup of the red cell causes clotting of the blood by starting the clotting process through activating Factor 8. By taking a known amount of red cells and bursting them by adding a small amount of distilled water, the researcher can have a controlled concentration of this factor. It has been named erythrocitin. To make a long story short, if using a substrate of plasma with no Factor 8 and adding erythrocitin, scientists can detect extremely small differences in the concentration of Factor 8 in a specimen of blood added to this mixture. By drawing blood from medical students coming out of lecture, we established the range of Factor 8 concentration in normal control subjects.

I would take test tubes containing anticoagulant, syringes and needles, and a pocketful of dollar bills down to the lecture hall. Waiting as the students came out, I would cry out like a street vendor, "Does anyone want to get paid a dollar for ten ccs of your blood?" I would return to the laboratory with tubes of blood, dirty syringes, and an empty dollar-pocket. What we found was the maternal carrier's Factor 8 blood levels were exactly one-half between the normal controls and the marked deficient levels of Factor 8 in the patients with hemophilia. We had a reliable test for hemophilia carriers.

We submitted the article to *The Journal of Clinical Investigation* for publication. After a period of time, the manuscript was returned to us because it had been turned down by the Reviewing Board. They sent along the board's critique for our perusal. There was only one disclaimer, a professor in a Carolina school who simply said he didn't believe it. We didn't dwell on it but submitted the same manuscript to *The Journal of Laboratory and Clinical Medicine*. It was accepted and published in a few months.

About two months later, the reviewer who just couldn't believe our work published an article in *The Journal of Clinical Investigation* with the very same findings as ours. It takes a certain amount of time to get your work published in a journal, even if you are one of the individuals on their review boards. I don't know whether he was already doing this work and he was trying to delay the publishing of our work, or whether he figured that we had really made a significant finding and he wanted to get it into print first. At any rate, he was second, and his attempted coup of our work served only to confirm our findings. I resisted the urge to write him and express our appreciation for his confirmation of our published work. Truly there is no honor among thieves, in spite of their academic accomplishments.

Every Friday, the university set up a seminar in the Mayo

auditorium where each department was responsible for providing a faculty member or fellow to present a paper on his or her ongoing research work. They served sandwiches and non-alcoholic drinks for the audience. Everyone attended this, and there was always a packed house. For this reason, there was great competition among the various departments to present something new and significant. I was picked to present my erythrocitin data for the department of pediatrics. I presented, and it was very well received. Later, when mulling over this experience, I wondered whether it was because they liked the work, or whether they just liked to hear me talk because of my southern accent.

During all the laboratory work I also had clinical duties and experiences. We had hematology and oncology clinic once a week. Of course, during any hospitalizations, we always were the consultants in hematology and oncology for the ward pediatric resident or, on some occasions, the admitting physician.

Some of these patients received "experimental" drugs, which meant that they had not been released by the FDA for public use. To use one of these drugs, application to the FDA was required, with explicit indications for its use clearly defined. We didn't participate in any large protocols, where a large group of patients were given either experimental drugs or a placebo (sugar pill) according to very specific rules. When we used such drugs, it was decided according to our own specifications.

I recall one little fellow who was about eight or nine months old. He had a large tumor which literally filled his chest and markedly restricted his breathing. A biopsy showed embryonic cells that gave no clue as to their organ of origin. We tried radiation, plus other chemotherapeutic drugs, to no avail. In a decision spurred by desperation we obtained permission to use five-fluorouracil IV, as this was an experimental drug at the time. The tumor disappeared in just two or three weeks and never returned. I've never had it work too well on anything else. Apparently this tumor consisted of cells in early development that could be kept from reproducing by inserting a fraudulent uracil to be used for the DNA production in that cell line. We didn't know what cells this tumor arose from, so we really didn't know why the drug worked so well, and we still don't. I've never seen another one, so I can't have a series of two that I can report and have it bear my name, i.e. Bentley's Tumor.

Another very good aspect in being among this pediatric faculty was that it always had prominent visitors. Whenever they dropped by, they were always asked to give a presentation on their work in progress. I guess they always expected this because they all brought slides. It was a magnificent learning experience.

Bob Good's research territory involved the whole top floor of the Variety Club Heart Hospital. This hospital was where all of the pediatric cardiology patients were cared for, and it was where the first successful heart-lung machine was conceptualized, built, and used. Because the hospital and Bob Good's chair, The Variety Club Professor of Pediatrics, were built and funded by donations from the Variety Club, we had actors always visiting for photo ops and other publicity. Usually they would show up with no advanced notice, with a photographer in tow, and some faculty would show them around.

One day, Gregory Peck, a very famous and distinguished actor at the time, showed up, and it so happened that none of the regulars were around. In the research area there were many PhD's working on immunology projects, and they were totally consumed by their work. The outside world was of no consequence to them. Well, this day only one of these gentlemen was available, and he was conscripted and sent out with Gregory Peck in tow. After several stops and innumerable pictures, this guide had run out of small talk, so he turned and politely asked, "Well, Mr. Peck, what type of work are you in?"

Bob was the second genius that I have ever known. He received his MD and PhD degrees the same day, both being awarded summa cum laude. His output of work was legendary, as was his work ethic. He would come to work about ten or eleven o'clock in the morning and would often work until two or three in the morning. His wife would call the lab and tell us, "You boys be sure that Bob remembers to eat." One such story that confirms his wife's concern occurred when Bob was sitting in Al Michaels's office discussing some experimental results. He kept looking at an apple sitting on Al's desk. Finally he said, "Al, would you mind if I have that apple; I can't remember whether I've eaten or not." Al would go on to become dean of the School of Medicine at the University of Minnesota.

Bob laid out the workings of the immune system, the thymus gland, T-cells, B-cells, etc. He started the Hagfish Society, which met every year at the Federation Meetings. It was a society for people working in immunology to get together to hash over new ideas, have discussions, and revitalize their excitement over new findings. The society was so named because the hagfish is the lowest form of animal life that has an immune system.

Bob had one of those faces that perpetually sagged. His eyebrows even angled down on the outer edges. He eventually left Minnesota and took the position of director of research at Sloan-Kettering Institute in New York City. After his appointment, his face was on the cover of *Time Magazine*. Afterward, he said that when people were featured on the cover of *Time*, they usually were flooded with congratulatory notes and letters from friends and colleagues. He claimed that all he received were six letters from plastic surgeons, offering to remove the circles from under his eyes.

Bob remained a good friend through the years. I always thought that he should have been awarded the Nobel Prize for his work on the immune system. He came down to visit several times and gave several lectures for me. He's now dead, but what I remember the most about Bob was when we talked on the phone, he would always start off with, "Herschel, it's so good to hear your voice."

As the days grew longer and slowly began to warm up to a high of thirty-two degrees, people began to venture forth into the daylight. The house that we rented was in a working-class neighborhood. Each Friday afternoon, residents would see men coming home from work with their round containers of beer after a stop by the local tavern on the way home. This was beer country, and everyone readied themselves for the weekend with stashes of beer. Each had a rather short, but large in diameter, canister with a bail handle, and the bartender would fill it with beer from the tap. No six-packs for these drinkers with Viking ancestry.

The improvement in the weather also meant that Paul could go outside to play. He had a small tricycle that he could pedal at amazing speed. We lived in the middle of the block, and he would pedal on the sidewalk down to the corner. He would stop there and watch whoever was outside with him very closely. As soon as anyone turned their head away from him for a second, he would pedal like mad on the side street sidewalk. This meant that his parents had to get up, walk down to the corner, and look. He usually could be found at the same place, and he got a lot of pleasure on making us walk down there. One day, Nancy was home alone with him, being even greater with child and watching Paul play on his tricycle. He pulled his same trick, but this time when she got down there Paul was nowhere to be found. After looking for him desperately, she really panicked and called the police. They came and found him pedaling up the alley that ran behind the house.

Paul was always doing things when I was away from the house. One day, I got home from work and leaned down and picked up Paul. When I got him to the level of my ear, I could hear him wheezing. I asked Nancy what was causing him to wheeze, and she said just before I got home he had picked up a pencil and bitten the eraser off before she could get it away from him. Well, it was obvious that he had aspirated the piece of eraser. I called poor Bill Krivit another time and met him at the University Hospital. After listening to his chest, he agreed that he sounded like he had a foreign body in his lung. He called an ENT colleague who came over immediately. Paul was taken to the operating room, and they got three small pieces of eraser out by bronchoscopy. He had to stay overnight for observation. This was my initial experience with hospital dictum, that no one was allowed to stay with a child while he or she was hospitalized. I was dumbfounded. The child had just been to surgery, and now his parents were abandoning him. At least that would be his perception of the entire affair. In the future that was yet to be, I would stop that practice wherever I had the authority. I picked him up the next morning, and he was very glad to see his old dad. Again Bill had come to my rescue.

The first summer that we were in Minneapolis, Nancy's folks came up to stay for a short visit. I knew that Claude Taylor would want to go fishing, and I began to ask around about where we could go and fish for bream. They call them "sunnies" up there. Several people recommended a lake up above Minneapolis. After they rested a little while from their two-day journey, we set out for the lake. Now, up there they don't fish for bream too much. They prefer to fish for the big ones like pike, muskies, etc. We found the lake and a place that rented boats.

We asked the boat renter where would be a good place to fish for "sunnies." After looking at us as if we had lost our minds, he reckoned that we might try to fish for them in some reeds growing off the northern shore. He didn't have motors to rent, but the boats were fitted with oars. These were large boats with oar locks in the center of the boat, not the small skiffs that we were accustomed to at home. You can guess who manned the oars, and though I had never done it before, we quickly made it over to the large reed beds. We had a system in our fishing. I sat on the stern with a canoe paddle and paddled, while C. T. cast small white popping bugs until we found them. We never seemed to vary from that routine for some reason.

We started fishing the edge of the reeds, and almost immediately C. T. got a strike. He tried to set the hook, but there was no fish there. This usually means that the fish was too small to be able to get the hook in his mouth. We kept fishing and getting strikes, but no fish. I kept giving him encouragement, such as, "If you are not going to catch these fish, I am going to let you paddle and I will catch the fish." This didn't seem to inspire him, however, and he kept casting. Suddenly he hung one. His fly rod bent double and it was obvious that he had a pretty good fish on there. After a short battle, he landed this huge bream. It had to weigh a pound and a half. Bream really fight when you hook them, and I have always said that if they grew as large as bass a fisherman would never land them.

When he landed that one, we both started fishing and landing huge bream. We continued until we began to think of the limit of the number of fish that we could keep. We looked it up in the little booklet that C.T. received when he got his out-of-state license. We found that between the two of us, we could keep about fifty bream. We quit when we got to that number and went back to the boat landing. The next day we returned and got another boat. When we looked over at the spot we had fished the day before, it was covered with ten to twelve boats, all fishing for bream with cane poles and worms. I rowed us over, and we resumed our fishing with small white popping bugs, just as we had the day before. We repeated our performance of the previous day. After a short while the discrepancy between the two methods became obvious. One of the guys in another boat yelled over, "What kind of fishing are you doing?"

C.T. yelled back, "Alabama style." We gave away all the catch for that day.

The next summer, Nancy's folks came back again, and C.T. and I went up to our lake once more. We went to our old spot but didn't catch a thing. We could not find one little bream to catch. It had rained a lot that spring, and it had changed the water level. We were disappointment personified.

During my first summer, I became aware of the obvious differences between the pediatric departments at Minnesota and

Alabama. The department at Alabama didn't demand, nor did it acquire, any esteem from others for the quality of faculty or of its academic programs. The faculty, as a rule, could be found in the main pediatric office sitting around drinking coffee, socializing with the departmental secretaries, making snide remarks about people walking down the sidewalk on 20th Street, or just being cute with house staff or drop-in visitors. There was no research of any consequence going on, no papers being written, nor any investigations of any sort being conducted.

The education program consisted of ward rounds, which concentrated solely on clinical diagnosis and current therapy. There rarely was any discussion of the pathologic state, what caused it, or why the therapeutic plan was selected. It had the aura of a trade school where the student is taught a trade and how to pursue it, and then the individual would not have any understanding of why anything changes in ten or so years. Usually such trained physicians resist change vigorously, or they hop onto every drug being hawked by a drug representative without any hope of understanding what exactly they are doing. Their excuse: "I just want to use the latest thing for my patients."

In contrast, the faculty members at Minnesota never were seen around the coffee pot. The entire faculty attended all the numerous teaching conferences; ward rounds were only attended by the house staff, students, and the attending faculty on the ward. Grand rounds were held every week, where interesting or puzzling patients were presented for the entire pediatric faculty to chime in and give depth to the discussion. No one was ever seen sitting around shooting the breeze. Faculty member and their fellows had numerous projects going on, and they were busy doing whatever that called for in order to get all the work done. It was all business-like and highly professional. Also, the house staff and fellows had an attitude of quiet confidence and pride in the teaching program, the faculty, and themselves. This contrast impressed me greatly, and unconsciously, I suppose I made a mental note of it.

That summer, as the pediatric faculty and fellows were sitting around the lunch table in the faculty dining room at the student union building, Lewis Wannemaker asked, "Does anyone here know how to lay brick?"

Well, do you remember my building our first garage/shop? I replied, "I do." And that simple question and answer was the beginning of a friendship with a very brilliant investigator and an extremely warm individual with a wonderful wife, Hallie. Lewis was a very quiet individual who always spoke in a quiet voice, and very seriously, about everything. He was one of the world's experts on the germ streptococcus. He also was a member of the team of investigators who discovered that rheumatic fever was caused by strep throat.

This request had to do with more mundane things, such as laying brick for a raised flower bed on his daughter's playhouse that he was building. I think, with some trepidation on his part, he invited Nancy and me over to his home one weekend to build the flower bed. It didn't turn out to be much of a job, but it did greatly enhance the looks of the house. It was built at the end of the little front porch. I helped him with a few other construction jobs before the house was ultimately finished. I truly think that he was surprised that I could lay a stretch of bricks that were level and didn't look like the bounding main.

Lewis was a devout gardener and was glad to find out that I liked to garden also. He always laid out his rows precisely, and he was absolutely adamant that the rows were perfectly aligned. He was always trying to raise sweet peas, but for some reason they just never did right for him. He came over to our place one summer day and discovered some absolutely gorgeous sweet peas that I planted in the spring by using a pick-ax to dig up the frozen ground. He was immediately seized with unbridled envy. Envy is one of the seven deadly sins, if you recall.

Lewis and Hallie took us under their wings during my fellowship. They had season tickets to the University Theatrical Program, which presented dramas, comedies, and musicals by the theater students. It was always very well done, and Lewis and Hallie always bought two extra season tickets for their guests. They shared them with us on many a joyful occasion.

Lewis had a habit of going to bed early and rising about four o'clock in the morning, which gave him quiet solitude to read, to study, or just to meditate on his research projects. He did this almost every day, and once he had gone to sleep in the evening there was no waking him up. Hallie had invited us over one night, and when we arrived we found that Lewis had fallen asleep on the couch. Hallie invited us in, and she was her usual graceful self. We chatted for a short while, until it was time to have dinner. Lewis was still softly snoring stretched out on the living room couch.

Hallie got up, took Lewis's table setting off the table, and invited us to join her at the dinner table. She said, "Oh, we'll just have to ignore Lewis; we wouldn't be able to wake him. He will just sleep there until about four in the morning." She was completely unperturbed by the entire incident. We had several similar episodes later on in our stay in the far North, and Hallie always found them amusing. Lewis died several years ago of a coronary occlusion, and I have always regretted that I didn't take the missed opportunities to thank him for being so kind to us while we were up there. He was a unique and wonderful person.

That fall, Paul Quie, one of Lewis's fellows and an alumnus of St. Olaf College, fixed it so that a bunch of us fellows and residents went down to St. Olaf and did physical exams on incoming freshmen students. It took a day, but they fed us and paid us very well for our labor. The money was a welcome addition to me, now with two babies to feed.

The next semester, I had to take a graduate class in biochemistry called Nucleic Acids and Protein Metabolism. I wasn't too thrilled about being required to take it, but it turned out to be the best course I have ever taken. It was taught by Dr. Cy Barnum, and it was the first course that I had ever taken that didn't require a textbook. The reason, apparently, was that the field was developing so rapidly that a textbook would be hopelessly outdated by the time it was published. Dr. Barnum would come into the lecture room and write four or five references in the literature that was the source for the day's lecture. Basically it was lectures on the formation of nucleic acids from purines and pyrimidines, and the DNA or RNA that were formed from the nucleic acid sequences.

I was having difficulty grasping the overall picture of the ultimate forming of chromosomes from these interactions when, one afternoon while I was going over lecture notes in the pediatric library, the entire picture just fell into place. From that time on, it was clear as crystal how the entire process occurred. Then chemotherapy became easy to understand and all the complications were just common sense results, not some list of side effects of drugs to be memorized.

The formation of a purine or a pyrimidine is a progression of chemical reactions to the final product. Physicians can use chemotherapy to block a step in the formation of these chemicals or substitute an altered purine as in 5-flurouracil or 6-mercaptopurine. As expected, the blocking of the formation in the early process of this formulation is a great deal more toxic, with more side effects, than that substitution of fraudulent pyrimidines or purines. Once I could visualize the big picture of all cell formation, be it normal or malignant, the entire body construction became clear to me. That knowledge was going to stand me in good stead later in my medical career.

I continued my clotting investigations into the chemical sequence that occurs from the beginning of the clotting process until fibrin, which is the head stuff in a clot, is formed. Fibrin is formed from a soluble protein in the blood stream named fibrinogen. This change occurs when thrombin acts on fibrinogen to alter it into fibrin.

Thrombin, in turn, is formed from prothrombin by a reaction with a substance called thromboplastin. This is formed in a waterfall sequence of several clotting factors to form the thromboplastin. First we perfected the technique of making thromboplastin from clotting factors in normal blood and concentrating it by ultracentrifugation in the cold. Early on, we were able to show that the thromboplastin activity was directly related to its phospholipids content. The higher activity was associated with high total phospholipids content and vice versa with lower activity.

At the end of my tenure at Minnesota, Bill helped me write a research grant request from the National Institutes of Health (NIH) for money to continue this work when I returned to Alabama. It was awarded and was waiting for me when I got back to Birmingham.

In the meantime, Bill Benton had come up to Minnesota to complete his pediatric residency after his tour of duty in the Army Medical Corps. He was finishing up and was considering going back to Alabama to do a neurology residency. Hugh Dillon was in the process of finishing his tour of duty in the Air Force and would go into practice in Montgomery, Alabama, with Bill Daniels (remember that name). Charlie Alford was finishing up his tour of duty in the Navy. I had decided that I was going back to Alabama to see if I couldn't help get the department on a little higher tone.

Nancy's folks came up, picked up the boys and her, and they headed back to Alabama. I stayed around until the movers had all of our belongings packed, and I then started the drive back South. I have never returned since then, though I have seen all my old friends at meetings through the years. It was a wonderful and educationally profitable time for me, and it changed how I looked at medicine forever. Now things were about to happen that I had never even considered before.

Chapter 9

Academia at Alabama — What Happened to My Lifelong Dream?

"If you want to make an enemy, change something."
— President Woodrow Wilson

I was given the appointment of assistant professor of pediatrics at the University of Alabama, with a salary of ten thousand dollars a year. It doesn't sound like much, but considering I was coming from a position paying thirty-six hundred dollars a year, it seemed like an awful lot of money to us. We found a very nice home to rent in Homewood, Alabama, where the yard was carved out of the side of a mountain. The front yard was small and built on an angle of about forty-five degrees. Then, there was a flattened area where the house stood, a backyard which was covered with paving stones, and after a short stone fence about three-feet high, the mountain continued its upward way almost straight up. The home was much bigger than the one in Minnesota, but then what wasn't? It was two stories, with the second story consisting of attic space. It housed two bedrooms with dormer windows and a bath. The first floor contained a master bedroom and bath, a dining room, living room, and kitchen. On the front of the left side of the house as one faced it was a one-car garage that never housed a car while we lived there. It was a great storage area, and I used it as a workshop. It was a very nice house and affordable as far as rent was concerned.

On our first day at our new home, we were unpacking boxes and the movers were placing furniture around in the various rooms when a distraught young lady in a station wagon drove up and parked in front of the house. She got out of her car and came toward the house carrying some type of bundle. I just assumed that she belonged to some welcoming committee such as Welcome Wagon. However, as she grew closer, I could see that the bundle was a very young baby, swaddled for warmth. She asked, "Are you Dr. Bentley?" I answered that I was, and she began to tell me that she had been waiting for me to get into town for quite a while. She had been told that her newborn child had some type of blood disease, and when I got to town she should take her to see me. We went inside the house and put the child on a table that was awaiting a place in the decorating scheme. I unwrapped the baby's clothing and took a look. The skin over the entire body was covered with grayish-blue infiltrates about the size of a match head. Nothing looks like that except neonatal leukemia. The gray-blue infiltrates are collections of malignant lymphocytes lying in the skin.

I didn't feel that I should tell her my presumptive diagnosis at that moment because that requires a very private area where parents have an unhurried moment to absorb such horrific news. I simply told her that it seemed as if her child did indeed have a blood disease, and I would meet her in the morning at the pediatric department for further testing. She came in, we confirmed the diagnosis, and I spent a very painful time delivering the news. It still had not gotten easier for me, but at least I was more skilled at it. That day, we started her on chemotherapy. Neonatal leukemia responds very well to treatment, and this child did also. She lived about eighteen months, which was about the average life span for treated leukemia in those days.

The Medical Center had changed somewhat since I had left to enter the Air Force. All of the area west of the hospital for ten blocks had been cleared under Housing and Urban Department (HUD) as slum renewal. Unfortunately, this also included the restaurant where all the medical students and house staff could afford to take their wives or dates to dinner. In addition to the University and Hillman Hospitals there were the Veterans Hospital, Crippled Children's Hospital, Spain Rehabilitation Hospital, and a new Children's Hospital under construction. The University Hospital and Children's

Hospital once again had separate residency programs, and the two entities were back on non-speaking terms. The University Hospital had secured a federal grant, and a state-of-the-art medical research unit for adults was being constructed on the third floor of the hospital. This was one of just a few such units funded around the country from NIH grant money.

I have a very strong suspicion that this grant was awarded mainly on political influence from Senator Hill rather than the quality and amount of research being done. I could easily be wrong, but I really don't remember any significant research coming out of that unit while I was there. I do remember their admitting a woman with a mass in her lower abdomen, and after an extensive investigation they found that her various hormone levels were markedly distorted. I don't know who the person was who finally figured out that the lady was pregnant.

A new building six stories high had been constructed and spanned 6th Avenue. It connected both the basic science building and Veterans Hospital on the south end with the University Hospital on the other end. Later this building would be named the Lyons-Harrison Building for Dr. Champ Lyons, the first head of surgery, and Dr. Tinsley Harrison, the first head of Internal Medicine. The building contained laboratories and offices for the various academic departments. The pediatric department was located on the fourth floor and claimed three-fourths of the space there. The remaining space was used by the neuroanatomy division of the anatomy department. This would be a fortunate happenstance in the years to come. I must explain my use of the term "claimed" to describe the pediatric department's use of its allotted space.

Things had not changed much in the pediatric department since my earlier departure. One faculty member had gone to join the faculty at Vanderbilt, and two female faculty members remained. Mac Bargeron, the pediatric cardiologist, was no longer in the pediatric department, but now he was a full time member of the surgery department. I never did learn what was behind all that. One of the remaining faculty members was in charge of the Outpatient Clinic, and the other was in charge of the Nurseries. I don't know who was in charge of the wards, but it seemed that the residents sort of ran it willy-nilly. I know when I started going down and looking at some hematology patients, they let me know they didn't appreciate my meddling with their patients. I very gently reminded them that they weren't their patients but the patients of the University, and they were allowed to participate in the care given as part of their educational program. See, already changing things, and I had just gotten there, Oh, well.

This new building had a large hall down the center, with laboratories perpendicular to the hall on one side and the staff offices down the other. After my experience with available laboratory space at Minnesota, this area looked like the expanses of the Gobi desert. The Department used very little of this space. They turned one area into a coffee area with tables, chairs, and a refrigerator. The only things that had changed from their previous quarters were now the windows were too small and too high to allow gazing down on pedestrians strolling below, and the secretaries were located across the hall in the Pediatric Department office. Thus they were left out of the banter that went on in the coffee room.

The really disturbing thing to me was the amount of time that the house staff and students rotating through pediatrics spent in this area just lolling around, joking, and being lazy. They certainly weren't taking care of their patients or learning any more about pediatrics. The "arrogance of ignorance" was in full sway. As the old adage states, "The more that things change the more they stay the same."

My NIH grant had been fully funded, so my time in the first year was mainly spent getting my laboratory set up. It is amazing how much minutiae has to be ordered, received, and put away. This included large pieces of laboratory equipment, such as refrigerated centrifuges, refrigerators, and deep freezes (both upright and chest type), to small items, such as a stop watch. It all finally arrived, and a certified laboratory technician was hired. The lab that I was assigned was huge. It had three lab benches, wall cabinets , regular benches, a working air hood, and a lot of space between the fixed items. It was far beyond anything than I would really ever need.

Since it was the only laboratory space that was being used, I suppose it was better to have someone busily employed there than in one of the smaller areas. The work that I began doing was to continue the work on the total amount of phospholipids present and its relation to the activity of generated thromboplastin. After we proved that fact, we needed to find which of the individually involved clotting factors needed in the act of generating thromboplastin were actually donating the specific phospholipids.

We injected dogs with radioactive phosphorous, and after a

period of time the dogs would be euthanized and their serum, plasma, and platelets would be separated. These things would then be put in test tubes, labeled, and flash frozen. All were stored in liquid nitrogen until they were used. Thromboplastin was generated by mixing the various needed clotting factors, but only a single one of the collected factors contained a radioactive factor. By using a different radioactive factor in each test we were able to show that most of the active phospholipids were derived from platelets, and some from serum. All of this was written and published. After we had this going for about one year, we began to work out exactly what phospholipids were being incorporated into the thromboplastin. We continued to work on this until other things took me away from this type of work.

I also began to get some of the medical students interested in various things that I was interested in besides my funded research. The pediatric residents were repeatedly admitting newborns that were born outside the hospital that were found to have extremely high levels of serum bilirubin. However, none of these babies showed any clinical signs of kernicterus (deaf, spastic babies). We began to wonder why they didn't develop brain damage, while children who had hemolytic anemia and hyperbilirubinemia as a newborn, frequently did develop this very specific brain damage.

What we established was when bilirubin is released into the blood stream, it is bound by the large serum protein albumin. This prevents it from entering the brain tissue because the combination is too large to cross the blood brain barrier. However, if bilirubin continues to be made it will eventually bind all the available albumin and the unbound bilirubin will go into the brain, where it is deposited in the basal ganglia, causing the condition called kernicterus. This information has been made superfluous with the development of the bili-light, but it was important in its day. This situation occurs because newborn children start tearing down their red cells immediately after birth. They are now breathing and don't need to have high hemoglobin levels to grab onto the oxygen that is carried to the baby through the placenta. The hemoglobin from the destroyed red cells is broken down in its degeneration into a yellow material called bilirubin. This results in elevated serum bilirubin levels, and the neonate deposits a great deal of that bilirubin in its skin. This makes the child's skin and the whites of the baby's eyes yellow, a condition called jaundice. If this child is exposed to sunlight or a fluorescent light, the bilirubin in the skin will be destroyed and thus the serum bilirubin is lowered as it refills the skin. The repetition of destruction and refilling will quickly result in a normal serum bilirubin level. It is considered routine nowadays to see newborns without clothing except for eye protection basking under a fluorescent lamp. This is the bili-light.

The student with whom I worked on this project eventually went to Minnesota for his pediatric training and took his pediatric infectious disease fellowship under Lewis Wannamaker. He is now on the pediatric faculty at Penn State University in Hershey, Pennsylvania. That wasn't too bad—one future pediatric faculty member recruited to pediatrics my first year.

In those days, subspecialists in pediatrics were as rare as hen's teeth. In short there just weren't any; when I arrived at Alabama, I was the only pediatric hematologist-oncologist in the South, except for Dr. Bill Thurmond over at Tulane. Since I was the only one in the South, it could be presumed that I would be overwhelmed with referral patients. However, it took a good while before the practicing pediatricians really believed that I had anything to offer. Gradually, I began to get referrals from around the area. Almost as an afterthought, I suddenly realized that maybe I should get some type of malpractice insurance. I talked with several people and it was almost a consensus that I could get it, but the likelihood of a suit was essentially nil. Since I was prescribing drugs that had multiple and disastrous side effects, I got a policy for ten thousand dollars. It doesn't even approach reality nowadays. At last, we had the pediatric hematology-oncology section up and running with an active research lab.

Somewhere along here, Bill Benton and Charlie Alford came back to the medical center. Bill was involved with his pediatric neurology residency, and Charlie was just trying to find something to do. He started out working with Dr. and Mrs. Hare in the measurement of total body water. They had gotten a new machine that was supposed to give data that would allow an investigator to calculate this. This would be very beneficial in their research work into the pituitary gland's control of total body water. To accomplish this, the new machine had to be calibrated. This was done by using bottles of various sizes and determining their total volume. It was a great deal easier to say than to do. When Charlie left to begin his virology fellowship, I don't think that he had ever been able to consistently produce data that could be reproduced.

Also around this time, Charlie and I began to tighten down on the quality of patient care on the wards. We began to require that the house staff be able to justify their treatment plans and laboratory work ordered. The day I walked in and found them dripping vitamins in an IV tube was the day I lost my cool. There were only three conditions associated with vitamin deficiency seen in those days. Two of these, scurvy and rickets, are treated orally, and vitamin B-12 deficiency (pernicious anemia) is seen very seldom in children—if it is seen, it is treated with intramuscular injections. This bordered on malpractice right there on a university teaching ward. We took the vitamins down and began to hold a tight rein on the residents' quality of patient care. I knew that we caused some people to be upset, particularly the individuals who had set up the quality controls previously in existence, i.e. the faculty that were there before we arrived.

During this time, one of the residents came to me and told me that the surgery department was having a conference on a treatment plan for one of the children on the ward. They planned to discuss this without any of the pediatric house staff or the pediatric teaching staff being present. Well, Charlie and I, accompanied by several pediatric residents, invited ourselves to the conference. The surgery attending faculty seemed surprised to see us, but I explained to them that since they were discussing one of our patients, we wanted to be part of the discussions. The attending surgeon seemed to be embarrassed by the entire thing and tried to assure us that we were welcome and needed. He explained that in the past, no one involved in the pediatric medical care had ever expressed a desire to be included. We had a good teaching discussion that was both friendly and fruitful. I thought I perceived the pediatric residents standing a little taller and walking more confidently as they left. Maybe we were beginning to develop some positive feelings from the house staff about this entire program.

During the late fall or early winter of that first year, I was elected to membership in the Society for Pediatric Research. This is a research society that meets yearly for several days for the presentation of new research work. It is limited to researchers in the pediatric field and individuals under forty years of age. The one for the older fellows is the American Society for Pediatric Research, and I was elected to that when I came of sufficient age. Because I continued to do research work after I left Minnesota, everyone thought that the work I had done since leaving Minnesota was good enough for my election. Bill Krivit nominated me and Bob Good seconded it. Now when I went to the research meetings, I could wear a name tag that said "Member." I believe that I am correct in saying that this was the first time a person from Alabama had been elected.

John Shackleford was a faculty member in the department of anatomy, and since he was about the same age as all of us, we began to have social happenings that included John and his wife. John was originally from Mobile, Alabama, where he grew up and was educated in the Catholic school system. According to his own account, John was apparently a wild youth. When he was in high school, he was in a car accident, hitting a telephone pole head on while speeding. He came out of this accident as a hemiplegic and has been confined to a wheelchair since then. However, it did sober him up, and he applied himself in school and became a fine anatomist.

He became a specialist in mucopolysaccharides, which are complex sugars that make up most of the mucous made in the body. The average individual is familiar with the mucous that is made in the lungs. This mucous is made throughout all of the lung tissue even to the microscopic level. That mucous rides on little hairs called cilia, and it rides them upward out of the lung. As it travels, it joins other tubes and the mucous amounts get larger and larger. Any fine contaminant in the air that is breathed into the lung is captured in this mucous lining that is slowly, painstakingly making its way up to the throat. There it is usually swallowed, but if there is a lot, it is coughed out. In infections of the lung such as bronchitis and pneumonia there is a great deal of mucous made. It is usually coughed up and spit out, which the individual refers to as sputum. Often the color of this mucous will identify the organism that is causing the illness. For instance, pneumococcus bacteria cause the coughed out sputum to be the color of iron rust. Likewise, tuberculosis causes it to be bloody.

John became an expert in the technique of identifying mucopolysaccharides microscopically with a technique called histochemistry. This is done by making microscopic slides of the mucous-containing tissue and identifying each mucopolysaccharide by the color it turned when stained with different reagents. This is where the paths of his research and one of my interests in a disease crossed. We were discussing cystic fibrosis one day, and John said

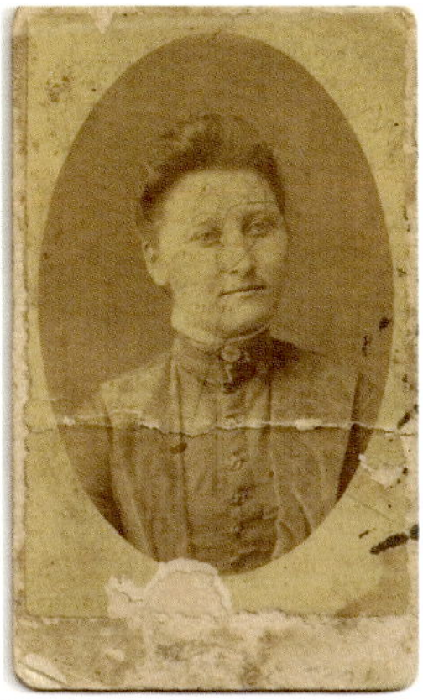
Grandmother Nancy Melverta Boozer

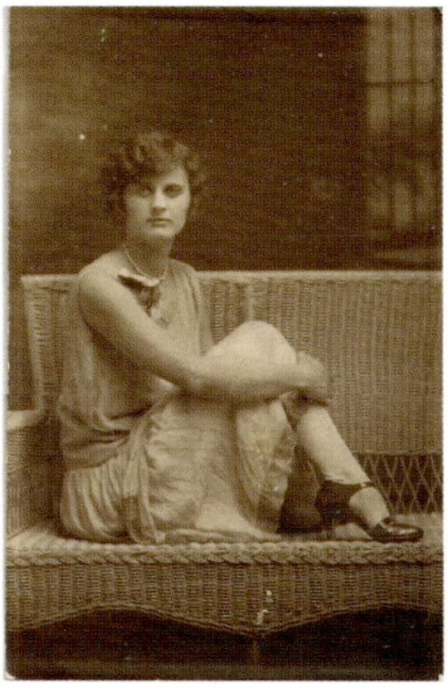
Mother, Frankie Mae Boozer Bentley

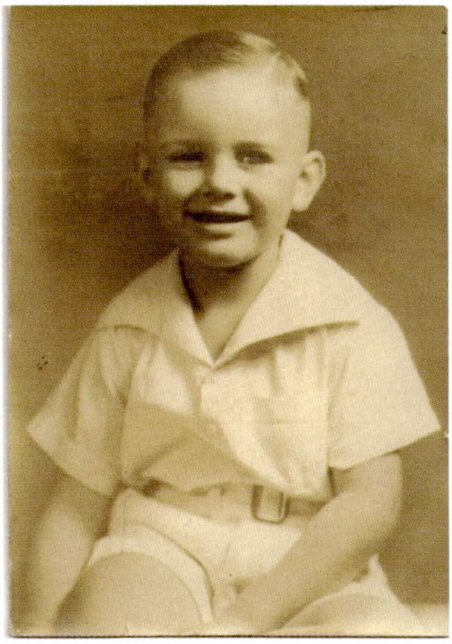
Herschel Bentley, about age 4

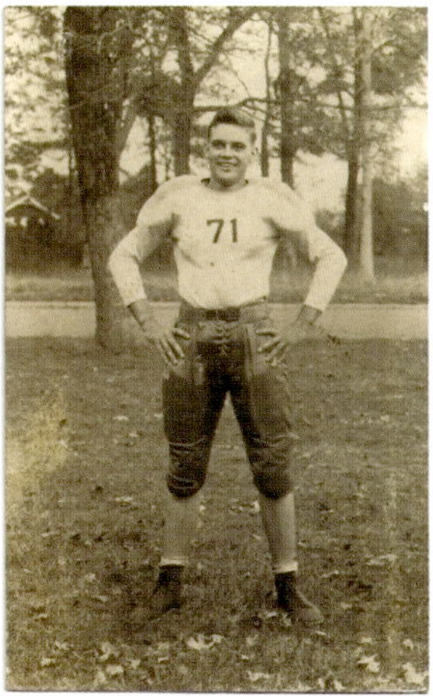

Herschel Bentley, senior, Amory High School

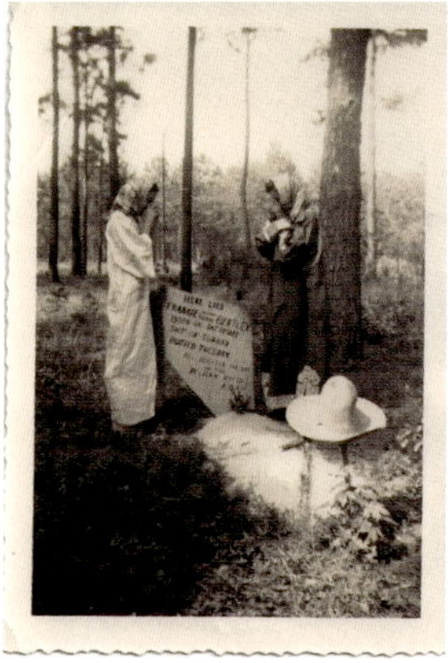
Funeral for the "dead man"

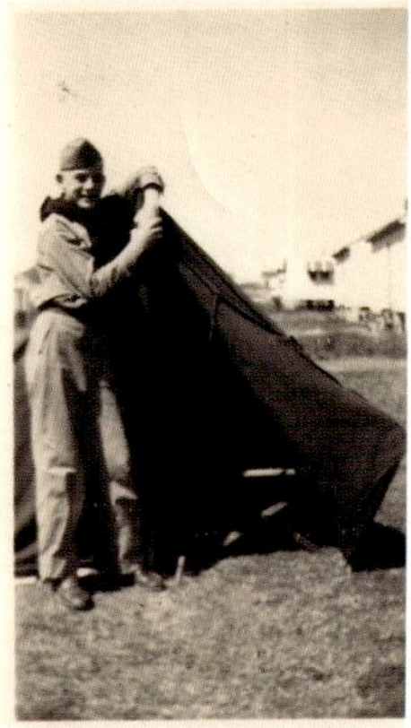
Eagle Scout Tom Bentley

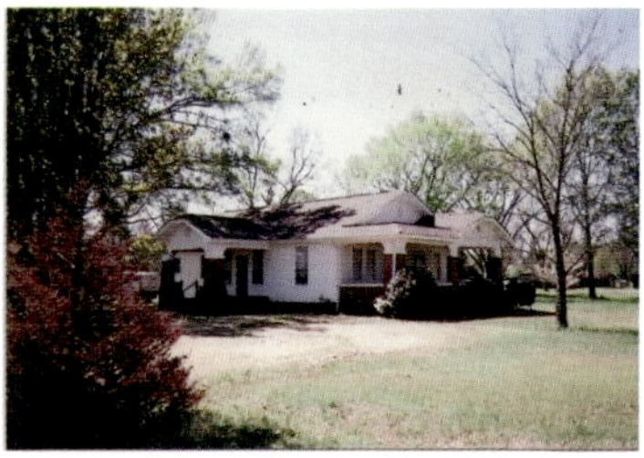
Grandfather Jerry Miah Bentley's house,
Amory, Mississippi

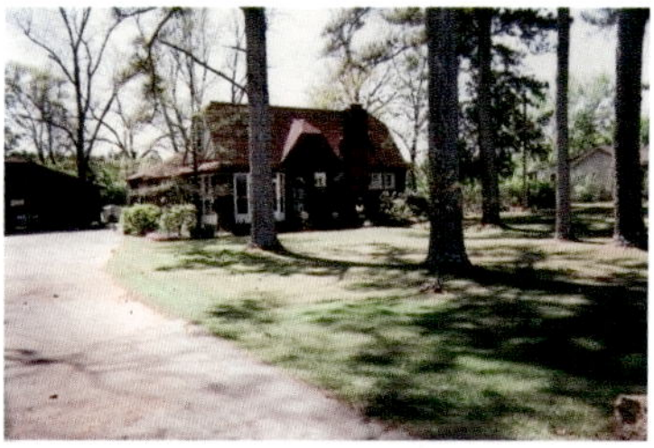
Childhood home until ninth grade,
Amory, Mississippi

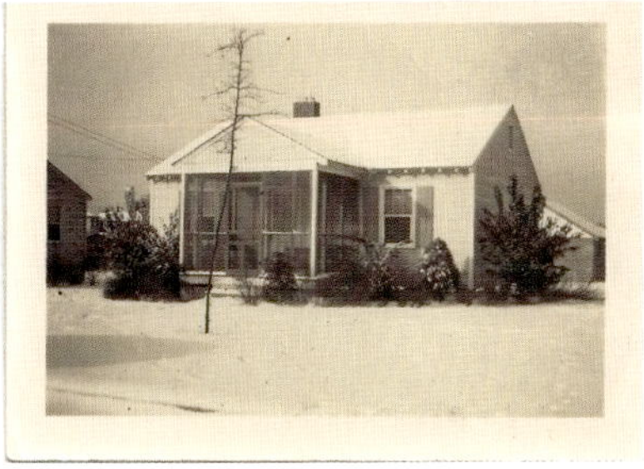

Gadsden, Alabama, house

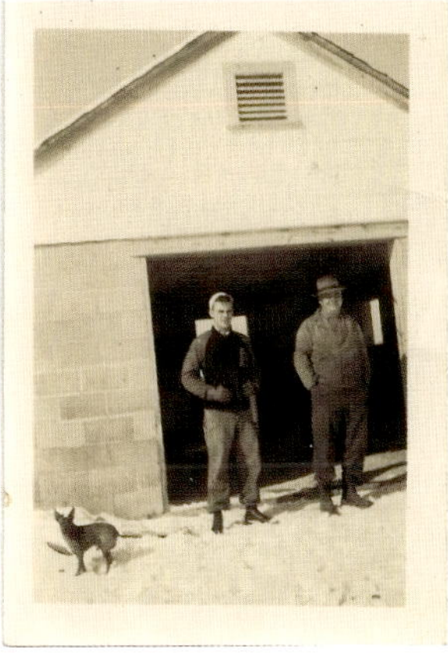

Hershel and his father at Gadsden house garage / workshop. Never had a car in it.

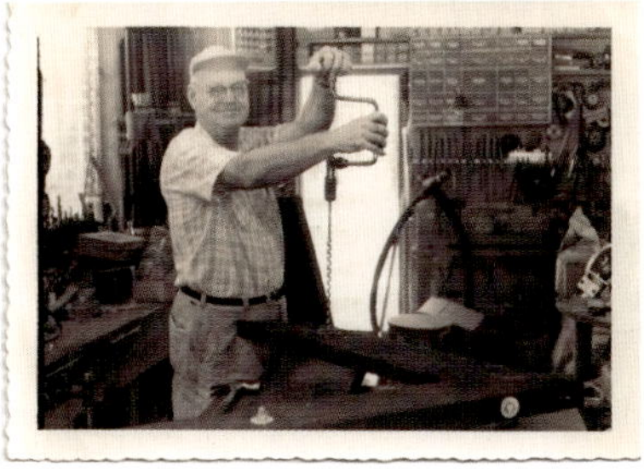

Herschel's father working on pier

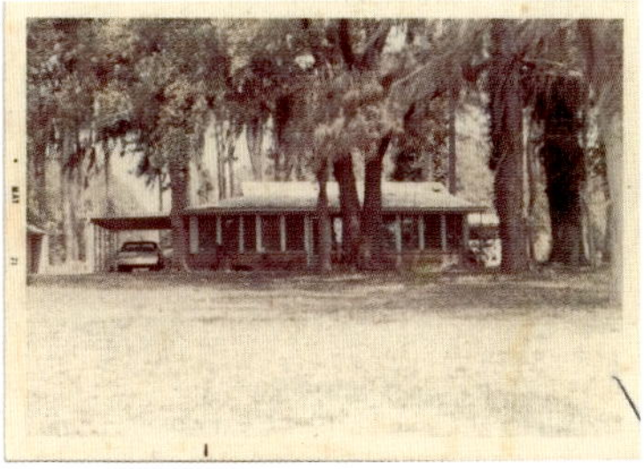

Baldwin County, Weeks Bay. "Dirt Dauber's Nest" built by Herschel's father.

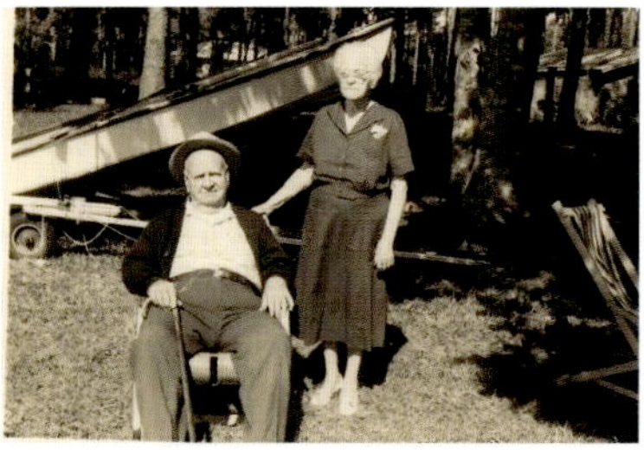

Grandparents Jerry Miah Bentley and
Connie Ethel Bentley

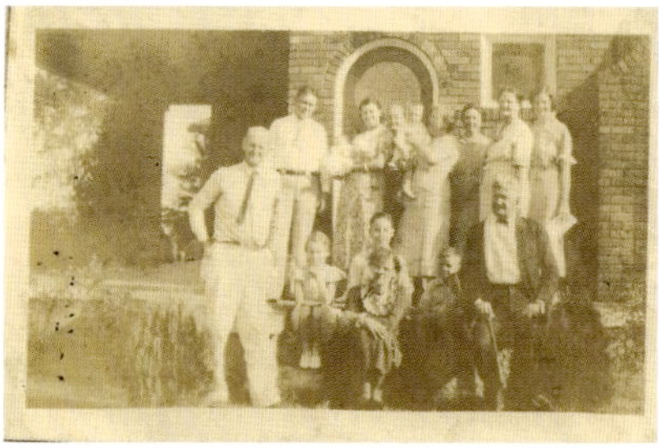

Clockwise from left: Grandfather James Presley Boozer, Uncle Robert Earl Bentley, Jean Bentley, Oleta Bentley, Dora Springer, Tom Bentley (in grandmother's arms), Grandmother Connie Bentley, and neighbors Mrs. Caldwell and daughter Rhee Caldwell, Tom Caldwell, Herschel Bentley, his mother Frankie Bentley, Uncle Jack Bentley, and Beth Brevard

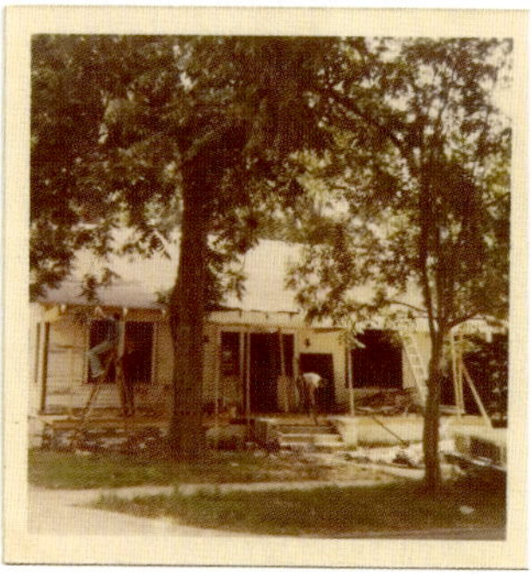

House on Texas Street: Before

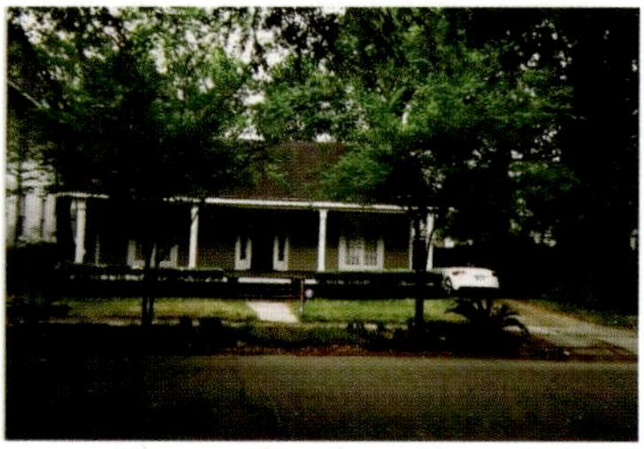

House on Texas Street: After

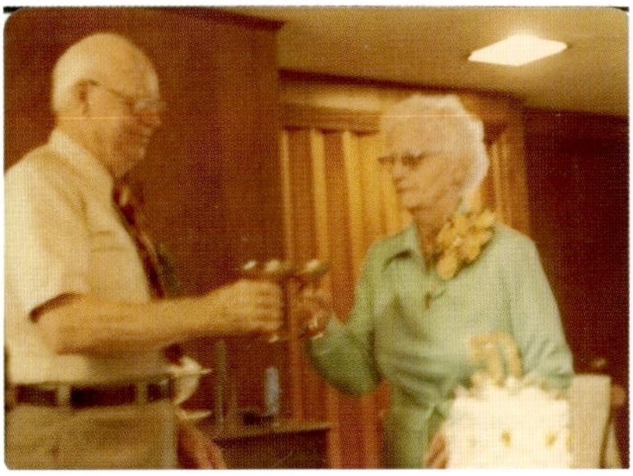

Herschel's parents at their 50th wedding anniversary

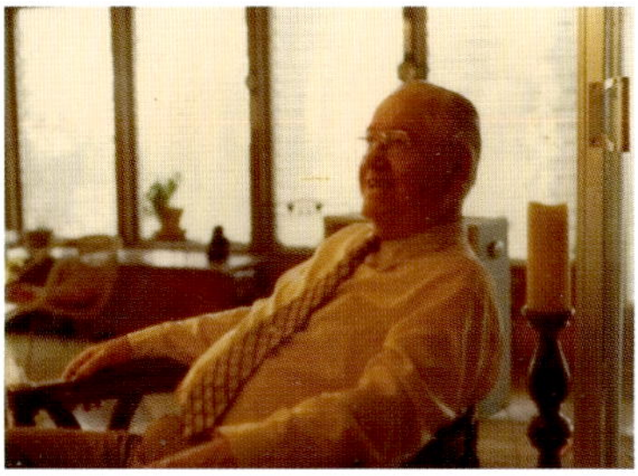

Herschel's uncle Marshall Bentley

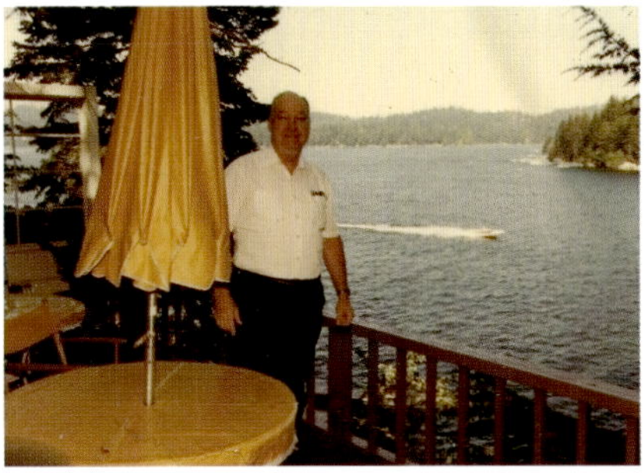

Herschel's youngest uncle, Jack Bentley

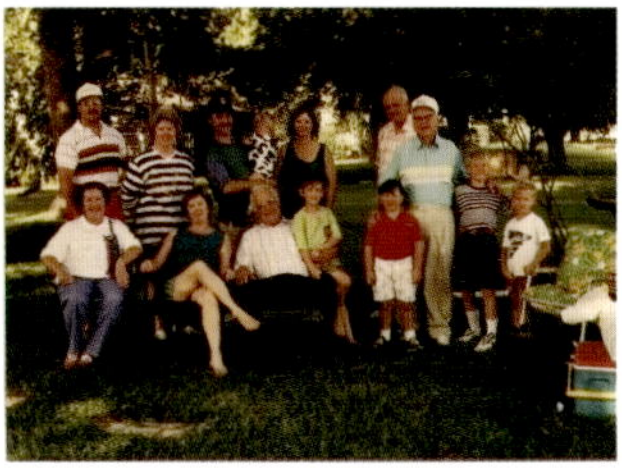

Herschel and Betty Bentley
with extended family

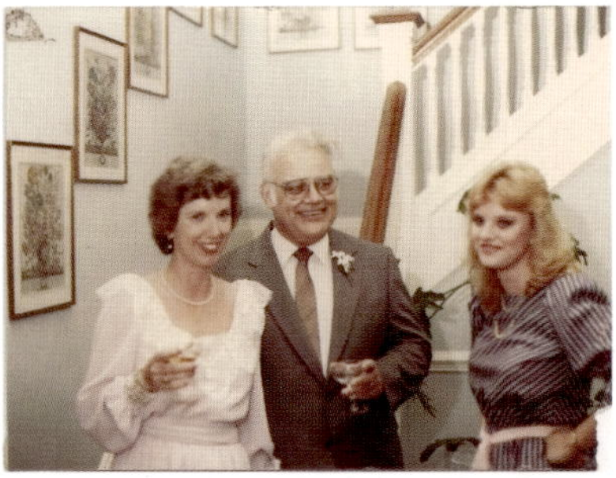

Herschel and Betty Bentley's wedding day,
October 22, 1983

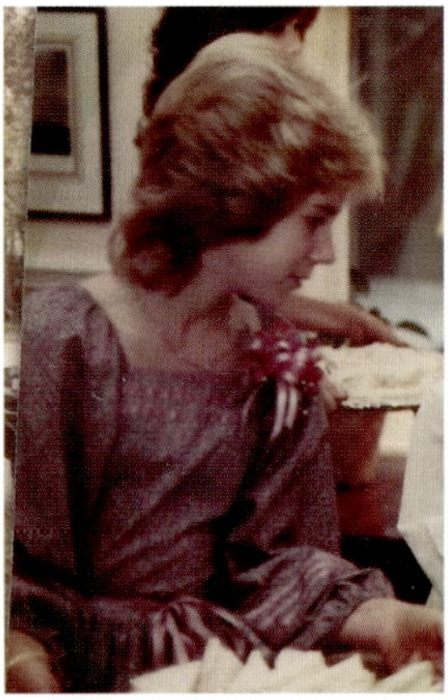

Abigail Parrish

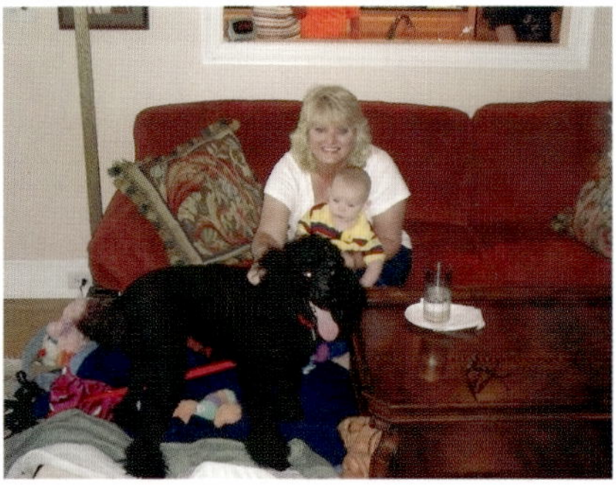

Daughter Valerie Pregeant, great-grandson Mark,
and dog Ellie

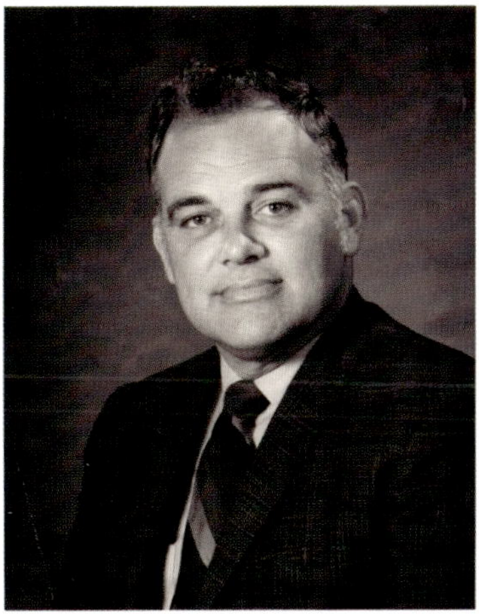

Herschel Bentley, M.D., Chairman of the Department of Pediatrics, UAB

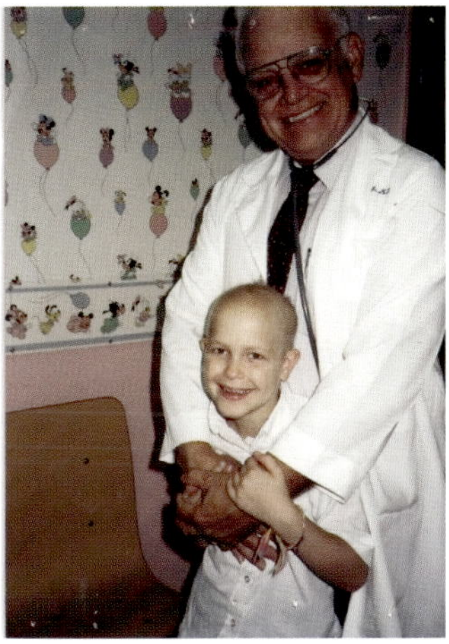

Dr. Bentley with a young patient

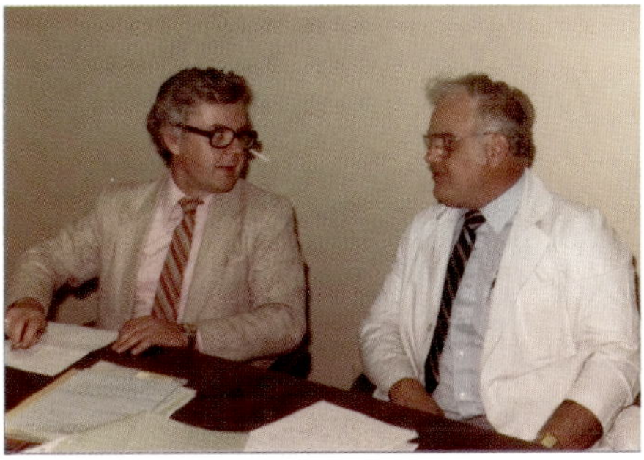

Wladimir Wertelecki and Dr. Bentley

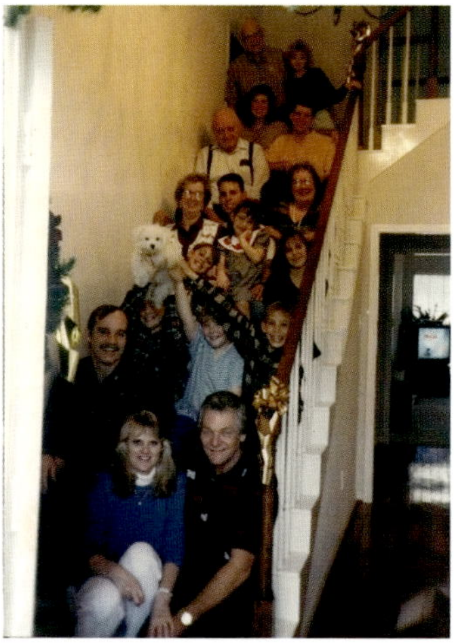

From top left: Herschel Bentley, Rhonda, Angela, Tom Bentley, John, Betty, Harrison, Jeannie, Megan Crawford (in Harrison's lap), Robert Crawford, Steven, Beck, Keith, Paul, Valerie, and Richard

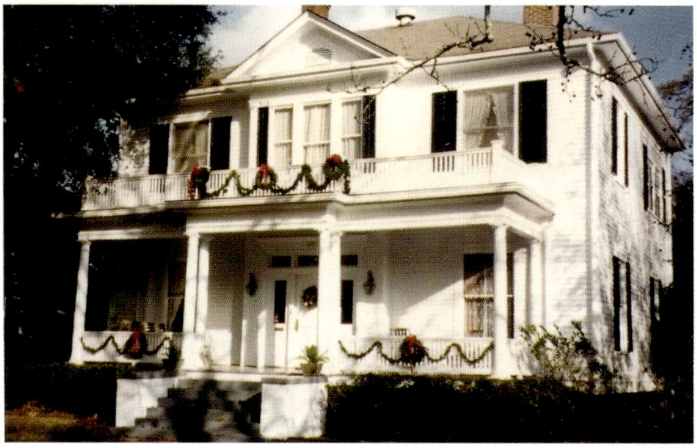

Selma Street house circa 1903

that he would like to study the mucous made in the lungs of patients with cystic fibrosis. The problem in children with this disease is that the mucous they make in their lungs and other organs, such as the pancreas, is so thick and sticky that it just plugs all the openings. John and I started haunting the autopsy room and gathered both normal and cystic fibrosis lung and pancreatic tissue for histochemical analysis. To make a long story short, we found that patients with cystic fibrosis inherit a gene that causes them to make all of the mucous produced in their body with the substitution of one normal mucopolysaccharide for a totally different one. This causes the patient to make mucous that is akin to chewing gum. This single change of one mucopolysaccharide alters the mucous in patients with cystic fibrosis so that it now repels water and is very thick and extremely sticky. Since it is an inherited condition and the child is just made that way, no effective treatment has been found. It is just going to have to wait on gene therapy or perhaps stem cell therapy to be cured. Gene therapy will be better because we can probably prevent its recurrence. The axiom is that it is better to prevent a disease than to have to treat it. Long ago we published these results.

We were beginning to get visitors like we did at Minnesota, but not in the same numbers. One day Dr. Bill Crosby from Walter Reid Army Hospital visited us. He and I were discussing sickle cell anemia. He was telling me about a guy who was admitted to his hospital with a painful sickle cell anemia crisis. They were doing the usual things for him, and the patient told them that the doctor in his hometown in the Caribbean would give him a shot of water in his vein and he would get immediate relief. Bill said that he told him the doctor was giving him water in the vein with the IV drip they had going and he said, "No, he just goes over to the sink, puts some tap water in a syringe, and gives it to me in one big shot in the vein."

He said they mulled it over for a while before they finally drew up 50 cc of distilled water and gave it to him in one big push. He quit hurting immediately. Bill said, "I'm not telling you to do it, but I am just relating our experience with this one patient."

It just so happened that we had a young boy on the ward in painful crisis. No one wanted to write the order, so I sat down with the boy and his mother and explained what we had just heard and that we wanted to try it on the boy's pain. After the mother gave her consent, we gave the distilled sterile water IV and he immediately quit hurting. Now this is no little pain that these people are having, but is gut-wrenching pain all over their bodies that causes grown men to cry. Since then, my residents and I have used it on numerous patients with good results. Many years ago we examined the data from these patients and have found that it always worked, except in patients who had received narcotics for the pain prior to receiving IV water. One of my residents and I published these findings about forty years ago.

There is also another condition seen in children with sickle cell anemia and who are usually under two years of age. They suddenly begin to scream with pain and to get significant swelling of the back of the feet and hands. The hands and feet rapidly become so painful that they scream if anyone just touches them. This is called "the hand and foot syndrome," and it occurs frequently in young babies with sickle cell anemia. This can be ended with the IV injection of 20 cc of sterile, distilled water. A hand or foot can immediately be squeezed without any demonstrable pain. The children are able simply to get up and walk out of the room. As one mother said to me, "Now, isn't that something?" To which I answered, "It sure is."

Sickle cell anemia is an inherited condition where the patient makes red cells that under certain conditions will assume the shape of a sickle, as in a hammer and sickle. The cause of this is the molecules of the red material in red cells, hemoglobin, will suddenly begin to stack one upon another and cause the red cell to assume the shape of the stacked molecules, which is a sickle. This slows down circulation of blood, causes clots filled with meshes of sickle cells to be formed, and leads to a drastic shortening of their life span. However, in true painful crisis there is no change in the circulating blood. There are no clots of sickle cells, or increase in anemia, and no changes in x-rays of the painful bones.

I began to think that the cause of painful crises may not be found in the red cells. The substance found in red cells that makes them red is a protein called hemoglobin. Its function in the body is to carry oxygen to the tissues. The redness is caused by an iron containing compound called heme. It is the thing that attaches oxygen to the hemoglobin molecule. The heme in turn is connected to a protein called globin, which is made up by a series of amino acids that are always identical. In sickle cell anemia, however, the sixth amino acid from the end of the amino series is changed. This causes the red cell to form a sickle shape, which in turn causes the very rapid breakdown of the red cells and extreme pain. The globin found in red cell hemoglobin and the globin of myoglobin, which is found in the muscles, has essentially the same amino acid sequence in their globin protein chain. What if the same alteration found in the amino acid sequence of sickle cell hemoglobin could also be demonstrated in the globin of myoglobin? Thus the pain in painful crisis could be due to the sickling of myoglobin in the muscle and nothing to do with the red cell. No one knows what IV distilled water does to myoglobin, but sickle cells are very resistant to hemolysis (red cell breakdown) in hypotonic solutions. I became so interested in this that I began to set up the techniques to study the amino acid sequence in myoglobin. We got to the point where we were able to separate myoglobin and start separating its constituents into component parts when other duties made me halt this work. As far as I know, no one has looked into this since I was working on it in the early 1960s. I am sure that the people with sickle cell anemia wish that someone would. Understanding the cause of an event leads to greater care for the patient and improvement in living pain free from inherited disease.

After a little over a year at Alabama, I came to the realization that things were not going to change there in spite of all my efforts. I've already explained the rarity of pediatric subspecialists in the United States, so opportunities weren't scarce. I accepted an invitation to visit the University of North Carolina to look at a position on its medical faculty. This was in October, when the leaves were beautiful with autumn colors throughout the heavily wooded campus. Everyone was extremely nice to me, and it was like something out of a movie. I came back home and thought about it for a while, and then Nancy and I drove back up there to let her see it. On the way up, I had a shooting pang of conscience and, after discussing it for almost the entire trip up to North Carolina, we came to the conclusion that I owed too much to the Medical School of Alabama to give up without trying a little longer and harder. We continued our trip, but I told Floyd after I returned home that I was going to stay put. That was the hardest decision I have ever made.

Later on that year, things had definitely not improved and one day I received a call from Dr. Ralph Platou, the longtime chairman of pediatrics at Tulane University. Dr. Platou was a legend in academic pediatric medicine, and at that time he had been chairman at Tulane for thirty years. He wore black horn-rimmed glasses, but as he pointed out to me, he didn't have any lens in one side. He informed me that he was blind in that eye, and he didn't wear a lens because if he were in an accident the lens might damage the cornea in that blind eye. Then, it wouldn't be available if it were needed for a corneal transplant in the future. He was always planning ahead.

We remained good friends for years, and I still have a book on trout fishing that he gave me from his private library. Although there was probably forty years' difference in our ages, we would always get together every year at the meeting of pediatric department chairmen and go on long walks together. We never discussed being a pediatric chairman a single time. He was just a straight-arrow type of guy; what you saw was what you got. He was indeed a wonderful person, and one whose friendship I cherished.

On this trip, Dr. Platou took me to dinner at Arnaud's Restaurant in the French Quarter. We parked the car and walked down the side of the building, and Dr. Platou rapped on an old, very sturdy-appearing door that, I was told, had been used by the bootleggers delivering booze during Prohibition. It was immediately opened, and we were escorted past a very busy kitchen into a small private dining room. We were seated, and a waiter just suddenly appeared at our table. Dr. Platou introduced me to the man who had been his sole waiter for thirty-three years. Needless to say, I enjoyed the attentive service and the great food immensely.

The next day led off with a meeting with Dr. Platou. We sat at his large, cluttered desk, and he opened the conversation with, "I believe that I should tell you something before we start our conversation about this position. I have been talking to several people up at Alabama, and they tell me that you are going to be offered the chairmanship of pediatrics in about a week."

I was totally flabbergasted and stammered, "Oh, I don't think so, Dr. Platou, I only finished my fellowship about a year ago, and I am only thirty-three years old."

He wasn't very impressed with my denial, and he continued, "Well, I know a lot of people up there, and they all tell me the same thing. If you do decide to take the job, I want to give you two pieces of advice that come from my thirty-plus years as a department chairman." He pointed to a stack of papers about two inches high sitting on the edge of his desk, "You see this stack of papers? I don't act on any complaints unless they are put in writing, and when they come in, I slip the complaint on the bottom of this stack of papers. By the time I get to it after taking care of the ones on top of it, it is amazing how many of those complaints have taken care of themselves before I get to them." He continued, "And the other thing that I want to tell you is, keep small things small." Those were, I believe, the best two pieces of advice that I have ever gotten.

We continued on the visit, and this matter was not discussed again except for one young fellow who said, "I hear that you are going to be offered the chairmanship at Alabama. I don't know, but it would seem to me that if you are good enough to be a chairman at the age of thirty-three, one would be waiting for you when you got older and had the chance to do some other things." I didn't respond to that other than shrug my shoulders, but it did give me something to think about.

I drove back over to pick up Nancy and the boys, who had been staying with my folks in Fairhope, Alabama, and we drove back to Birmingham the next day. We discussed what I had been told, but neither of us really thought that it was going to happen.

When I got back to work, everything seemed like it was before I left. It remained that way for about a week, and I was trying to decide about Tulane. The department secretary walked into my lab where I was working and she said, "The dean's secretary just called and wants to know if you would come down to the dean's office for a few minutes."

I said, "Tell her that I will be right down." S. Richardson (Dick) Hill was the relatively new dean of the school of medicine, and prior to this appointment, was professor of medicine and head of the endocrinology division in that department. He was installed as dean of the school of medicine at the same time that Joe Volker was appointed as vice president for health affairs. Dick was a big man with a very loud laugh and usually sat at his desk leaning back in his desk chair, so that he was sitting with the end of his spine in the chair seat and the heels of his feet on the desktop. I entered his office, and he greeted me cordially and asked me to have a seat.

He got right to the point of the visit and said, "You know, Herschel, the pediatric department has been in a mess for a long time. It has a lot of problems, and they appear never to change or go away. We have asked Dr. Hare to resign his chairmanship, and he has done so. He has also elected to retire immediately. We have had a search committee working for a while now, and they have recommended you for the position."

I sat there for a few minutes and said nothing. Though I had been warned that this was going to happen, I really had not made a decision about what to say if it were really offered. I realized that my days as a researcher would be over, even though I could try and continue. This wasn't the life I had picked out for my family and me, and it surely did away with my starting a practice in a small town.

Dick continued, "We need someone to take on this task, and if you don't take it we may be a long time filling this position, with further deterioration of the department."

I suddenly developed a very calm feeling about this entire thing, and I said, "All right." I really drove a hard bargain. I didn't even ask what my salary was going to be or what the budget for the department was. Dick simply said, "OK, let's get some people in here." With that, he lifted the phone and told his secretary to send everyone in. In came the press from newspapers and TV. The announcement was made, and then it was all over. Dick chose to wait until the next day to inform the pediatric faculty. Of course, he realized that they would read about it in the evening papers.

I walked out of the office, spoke to the secretary out of courtesy, caught the elevator to the fourth floor, and went into my lab and sat on a stool. I felt sort of numb and was just looking around at all my experimental work that I was giving up to do something I had absolutely zero experience in doing. At that moment in time, I suddenly felt very insecure in my decision. However, that quickly left me, and just as suddenly I felt very calm and collected about the whole thing. I never had any more qualms about my being able to do my job; I just had to decide how to make it work.

Many years later I would realize that I was in a situation very much like that of Pope John Paul II when he was made bishop of Krakow during the German occupation of Poland. He asked the cardinal who had informed him of his selection as the new bishop, "Pardon me, your Excellency, can you tell me why I was selected, since I am so young and inexperienced?"

The cardinal replied, "We couldn't get anyone else to take it."

John Paul said, "Oh."

The next morning, of course, everyone knew all about it. Dr. Hare was not there, and I never saw him again. Charlie and Bill dropped in to say how great they thought it was. When I talked with the ladies in the department, it was a totally different matter. I must say that their attitudes took me aback. I was taught that for every job there was a boss, and, like it or not, you did what he said to do with a smile or you quit your job and got out of the way. These women didn't have the same teacher. First, they let me know that, in their eyes, I was just a little lower than a snake's belly for undercutting Dr. Hare in his position, and they planned to stay on as faculty members but they were going to make my life miserable. Well, so much for the spirit of cooperation. I tell you one thing, they kept their word. If you want to know why I didn't just fire them; they had tenure, the scourge of any school's administration.

After the meetings, I sat down and just took stock. I had three faculty members other than myself in the department. Two of them hated my guts for accepting the job and for instituting the changes they knew were coming. The other one didn't have anything to do. Since Dr. Hare had left, no one else had any interest in the volume of bottles that Charlie had spent so much time in striving to measure. I immediately thought of the house staff, because the department would grind to a halt without house staff to do the routines of patient care.

I went to talk with the pediatric chief resident, Dr. Harry Register. Harry was an ex-Marine sergeant, and he was a year older than I was. He told me not to worry about the house staff; they were all relieved to have the change and expected that the teaching program would be improved. If at any time anyone needed an ex-Marine sergeant to run the house staff, it was now. Harry completely took the house staff worries off my hands, and I have told him many times that I couldn't have done it without him.

I can't remember the time sequence here, but at some time or other I called my friend Hugh Dillon down in Montgomery. I told him about the things going on, and I asked him if he would want to think about going back to Minnesota and doing a fellowship with Lewis Wannamaker. He could join me at Alabama when he finished and take care of the bacterial infectious disease teaching program. As I recall, he didn't hesitate, groan, or shout at me, but instead said "I'll talk it over with Lil (his wife.)." In no time he resigned from his practice affiliation, moved the family back up to frigid Minnesota, and soon became the country's expert on streptococcal enzymes and the body's response to them. That gave me one position potentially filled with a pediatric subspecialty.

I then decided I had to deal with the problem of the pediatric cardiologist being in the surgery department. I went over and talked with Mac Bargeron about my thoughts. He agreed with me totally, and in a short period of time we had Mac back in the department. That gave us two subspecialists in the department, and one in the hatchery.

I realized that I now had to establish some long-range plans so people would know what our dreams were for the future of the department and where the department of pediatrics was going to fit into the large scheme of medicine in the university and the state of Alabama. This included how we were we going to function as a department in the school of medicine and the hospital; how we planned to provide for the care of patients (both referrals and indigent patients from the clinic); and our plan to fulfill the pediatric referral needs of the state and raise the department's research and teaching standards so we were on the same tier of faculty competence as other exceptional departments in the world.

It seemed to me at the time that the best way to approach this was to take a long look at the big picture first, so as to understand the entire future picture and then work my way down. In order to be on a par with the big guys, we had to have an exceptional faculty. I learned this from the time I spent in Minnesota. This did not mean that we had to start trying to hire faculty from universities where they were ensconced, but I thought it would be far easier and more doable to identify bright young men or women who had the ability and inner drive to become one of the best. This meant that we were going to miss on some, but also we would truly score on others. We would use this faculty to educate superbly trained pediatric residents and eventually, fellows. The medical students would need to be taught pediatrics so they understood the changes that were bound to occur in the future. This was going to require that the student be given a very intense two-month course in pediatrics with wide exposure to a large variety of diseases.

Likewise, the faculty had to be deeply involved in research projects and must extend this research into superior patient care. After all, research is the teacher of the teacher. Otherwise, a doctor gaining all his or her knowledge from reading journals becomes a follower, not a leader. Our faculty had to be leaders. We weren't going to spend a lot of time teaching about formulas, breast feeding or other mundane subjects that pediatrics had dwelt on in the past. After all, breast feeding is the method designed to feed children, otherwise women wouldn't have breasts. Formula feeding is obviously a way to feed babies that is working very well. There is no reason to spend an inordinate amount of time on such subjects. Remember, we must "keep small things small."

We had to serve the state's needs by producing a steady flow of well educated students and pediatricians. This also meant that we had to provide the means to keep our practicing physicians educated on the latest findings in pediatrics and to provide the plan for, and the creation of, regional medical facilities with high-tech hospitals and clinics. The most obvious at that moment was the creation and staffing of regional intensive care neonatal units scattered around the state on a regional care basis. Intensive care nurseries were just beginning to be set up in hospitals to deal with the myriad of maladies that could befall a prematurely born infant.

At this time, premature infants were mostly placed in isolettes or incubators and otherwise left alone. The health care staff had to control the ambient oxygen level, for too much oxygen would cause retrolental fibroplasia and resulting blindness. In the research conducted in the few high-tech intensive care nurseries around the world, doctors were experimenting with arterial oxygen electrodes to accurately monitor oxygen levels in the premature neonate. We were far from this level of care, and there were neither plans nor money to do anything differently. Therefore, we must find a way to upgrade our newborn nurseries and simultaneously increase the intensity of our neonatology educational programs to include fellows. To do all of that we were going to need a neonatologist to set up the intensive newborn care nurseries and train the nursery staff to become a capable and efficient nursing staff. Neonatologists at that time were essentially unobtainable. That was just another little problem I had to deal with.

In order to teach pediatrics, the instructor must have an abundance of patient material that is not solely acute illnesses and emergencies. I was once told by a physician that he didn't like pediatrics because it was a specialty of epidemics and emergencies. We had to do something about that mindset. Though that is a vital part of pediatric education, the physician also has to be exposed to diagnostic dilemmas in order to know how to approach them. Pediatricians shouldn't have to refer patients just because they are out of the routine, but they should know how to approach these patients and treat them. A doctor must remember that referring a child to an adult specialist is never the proper approach. Adult physicians always think in terms of degeneration, while in pediatricians have to think in terms of growth and development. It is very similar to comparing a small new car to an old deteriorating limousine and thinking their problems are going to be the same.

We did have the indigent patients who occasionally supplied us with a chronic medical problem to teach from, but more often they would supply us with the acute care problems. These teaching patients should only be treated with the best of care, not just what we can do with the inadequate facilities we presently were required to use. Students at any level remember how a patient was cared for while they are watching or performing. They never seem to hear the disclaimer that if we had the means, we would be doing so and so. They seem to only remember what was actually done to and for the patient.

Therefore, all patients admitted to this service absolutely had to receive only the best of care, regardless of the source of payment. The quality of the faculty should allow the development of a very active referral service, and grow steadily as we added high-quality faculty members. Now the problems we had were how to finance all of this, to identify and successfully recruit new faculty, and to immediately start thinking about growing larger. It cannot be said that I dreamed small dreams.

Now you are going to accompany me on the journey that we took to accomplish all of this. I had more fun doing this than anything I have ever done.

Chapter 10

Hang On! — Things Are Changing

Before I was made chairman, another little snag appeared in the smooth waters. Children's Hospital had hired someone to become hospital director in the new hospital being built on the medical center campus. Harry Shirkey was the fellow's name, and he had been brought in from Cincinnati, Ohio, where he had a private practice in pediatrics. He considered himself a pediatric pharmacologist, whatever that is, and he intended to have a pediatric residency at Children's. That meant that our residents were going to be unable to access some great patient material. Essentially all of the sick children who were not indigent were admitted to that hospital. We were going to have to do something about that, but just exactly what I didn't know at the time. Right then it was more of a nuisance than anything.

I decided to tackle the education of the practicing physician first. What better way to announce the changes that were occurring at the University than to teach a postgraduate course each year that involved some specialty area we wanted to introduce to the medical community? We decided to have the course in early spring, when the weather shouldn't be bad, but before the various national scientific meetings occurred. I thought we should have the first course on pediatric hematology-oncology. I chose this not because it was my subspecialty, but it was an area in which I personally knew some people who could serve as the visiting faculty.

When we had made the decision to do this, we invited Bill Krivit and Bob Good from Minnesota and Nathan Smith, professor and chairman of pediatrics, University of Wisconsin. Nate's claim to fame was that he took care of Red Skelton's son when he developed leukemia. Nate also had a keen sense of humor and would help keep the mood lighter. For instance, he told the story about a fellow who was driving through rural Wisconsin and began to see a series of signs advertising a restaurant that apparently was on the road ahead. The signs kept repeating that this restaurant could make any kind of sandwich that a patron might want. This theme was repeated over and over so, when he saw the restaurant ahead, he drove in and parked. He strolled in and sat down on a stool at the counter, and he was quickly greeted by a waiter who said, "What may I do for you, sir?"

The driver said, "I want an elephant-ear sandwich."

The waiter replied, "I'll be back shortly." With that, he turned and went toward the back of the building. After a long while he returned and said, "I am sorry sir, but we are not going to be able to prepare that sandwich for you."

The driver smirked and said, "Couldn't find any elephant ears, huh?"

To this, the waiter replied, "Oh no sir, it's just that we have run out of those big buns."

We had our visiting faculty, we had an auditorium, and we were ready to present the first postgraduate continuing education course by the University of Alabama. I don't remember how I financed this thing, but we did charge a nominal fee. The program was well received, and the auditorium was filled for every session. It was a huge success, and it was a good beginning to a feature that would be repeated every year. Eventually, the university sat up a postgraduate continuing education program for the medical school, and we were relieved of being responsible for these individual courses in the future.

While these professors were visiting, Harry Shirkey kept insisting that they come two blocks down the street and walk through the ongoing construction of the new Children's Hospital. After looking at halls where patient rooms were to be built and other things that would be used for patient care, the group was very polite but obviously bored.

Finally, Bob Good said, "Where are your research labs?" The others began to pick up on this theme, and the tour ended shortly thereafter. Later on, three small research labs were added in the basement, with no idea what was going to be put in them.

Just after the postgraduate course, Charlie came to see me and said he thought that he knew what he wanted to do in his future. He thought that he wanted to work in infectious disease in virology. He really didn't know where he should apply for such training. Well, I certainly didn't know the answer to that one, so I suggested that we get someone to give us some advice on the matter. I called Dr. Floyd Denny at North Carolina, a cohort with Lewis Wannamaker in the strep throat studies under Ramelkamp and an excellent person specializing in infectious disease. We made arrangements for all of us to meet him at the pediatric research meetings in Atlantic City in two or three weeks. We met in Floyd's hotel room, and after introductions and the goal of the meeting was reviewed, Eliyah Ayoub, my Lebanese friend from Minnesota days, and I went to see *Pillow Talk* with Doris Day and Rock Hudson.

After the movie ended, we returned to Floyd's hotel room to find that they had worked out all of Charlie's future and had already made the arrangements. Charlie was going up to Harvard in a few weeks to start a virology fellowship with a Nobel Prize winner. He would train with one of a trio of pediatric virologists who won the Nobel Prize for growing the measles virus. They were now working on the Rubella (German measles) virus, and Charlie was expected to be right in the midst of it. Now, I potentially had my fourth subspecialist and had the infectious disease section well underway.

In the meantime, we were expanding our teaching program. Conferences on patients, grand rounds, and lectures were all part of the routine day, and the entire pediatric faculty was expected to attend all scheduled conferences unless some urgent matter prevented it. This only amounted to about an hour a day or less. Still, one day I felt compelled to rise before the beginning of a scheduled presentation by a pediatric resident and castigate the attendees for strolling into the conference late. I reminded them that the resident had put in many hours of preparation for the conference, and it was only common courtesy to recognize that fact. They needed to arrive on time, rather than to stroll in during the first ten minutes, thus interrupting the flow of the presentation. I will confess to being more than a little steamed at the time, but we had no more tardiness after that. The chief resident, the old Marine, gave me a wry smile and a thumb's up.

Things were looking up slightly, but we were working with a thin labor force. This was especially true since Charlie was up at Harvard. The future looked a little brighter, since Hugh would be coming down before long. At about the time of these musings Bill Benton strolled into the office. He sat down and bemoaned the fact that his neurology residency was not giving him what he needed to become a pediatric neurologist. We chatted for a while, and then I suggested that I could call Phil Dodge up at Massachusetts General, and see if he could come to Harvard to finish his pediatric neurology residency. I don't really remember how Phil and I became friends, but he used to call me all the time after he went to Washington University in St. Louis to be pediatric chairman and we would commiserate over the difficulty in finding good pediatric faculty. At any rate, I gave him a call and told him about Bill, his background, and his need to finish his neurology in a training program that was slanted toward pediatrics. He didn't hesitate and said to send him on up. I just turned the phone over to Bill and they got everything arranged. Now I had five subspecialists, although two of them were still in the incubator.

In the meantime, Hugh came back home and we got him installed in his office and laboratory. It was great to have a stalwart soul like Hugh at my side. It certainly helped to have someone working totally on my side. Mac was around, but he was so busy that he didn't have the time or the inclination to get involved in departmental squabbling. Hugh, however, was always quick to back me up, protect our dream, and join in the resistance to prevent other departments from trying to overrun us. I slept better at night.

I really wanted to add an endocrinologist to our faculty. It was a glaring hole in our teaching program. We all tried to do the job, but we needed someone who understood all these hormones in depth. I called Charlie, who was working out of Boston Children's Hospital with all the Harvard pediatric crew. I asked him if there was anyone finishing up a pediatric endocrinology program that we might want to look at. He gave me a name, Russell Cunningham, and I immediately gave him a call. I gave him a synopsis of what we were trying to do, what parts we had been able to accomplish, and what we were trying to do immediately. I invited him down for a look, and he accepted.

He flew in one early evening after it had gotten dark in Birmingham, which was fortunate because Birmingham was far prettier at night with all the lights sparkling than it was during the day when all the steel mill's smog covered everything. This could easily be seen from the air, and it would cause immediate concern about landing and breathing that thick, yellow smog. The thought and concern had occurred to me many times when flying into the airport. At night, the smog made the lights twinkle brightly. His plane arrived, and the passengers began to walk down the exit ramp. I didn't know Russ and had no idea what to expect. I reminded myself that I was looking for a Harvard man, so I needed to look for someone who looked like they were from Harvard. There weren't that many people debarking, so I didn't have too many choices.

Suddenly I saw a tall, thin guy who was wearing a rumpled tweed jacket, very narrow black tie, a buttoned-down, white shirt and thin legged pants with no creases. His hair was straw-colored and seemed to be totally unmanageable, with small whirls going off in all directions. He was just ambling along and looked as if he had just been awakened. I said to myself, this has got to be the guy. I went up to him and said, "Are you Russell Cunningham,?" He nodded that he was. Russ spent two days with us, talked to everyone, listened to our dreams. We made him an offer, and he accepted on the spot. Now I had six, four of us with a subspecialty.

Every week, the departmental chairmen got a piece of blue paper from the dean's office, which was printed on front and back. It detailed all of the different programs being offered around America and any grants being offered by foundations or the federal government. I usually went back to the office after I'd had supper and the kids had calmed down, and I'd spend n hour or so doing paperwork. While it was quiet I read all my mail, did all my dictation, and concentrated on my work without interruptions.

I was scanning the blue sheet one night when I came across an announcement about grants being offered to health departments to set up a program for pregnant adolescent girls and their offspring. I had the immediate thought that this might be the way to get some money for my nursery programs. I dictated a short note to the dean, told him about what I had just found, and asked what he thought about looking into it. I got a memo in reply saying to give it a go. However, it was only available to public health departments, and there didn't appear to be any way around that. So I went over to the Jefferson County Public Health Department, which was located only a block away across a parking lot, and had a chat with the public health officer.

I put my plan to him, which was that the grant would be granted to the health department, and there would be a contract between University Hospital and the health department as to the management of the funds. The health department would pay University a lump sum for salaries obtained through the grant. This would include the salary for the obstetrical director, who would also be a member of the obstetrics department and salaries for a neonatologist, assistants, nurses, etc., for the neonatal program. The personnel and all hospital facilities for the grant would be housed in University Hospital. The grant would pay rent on a monthly basis to University for the space occupied by the grant personnel, and this would be used to pay off a loan obtained by University to pay for the construction of neonatal nurseries and obstetrical delivery areas. The details of the money involved, and how everyone would be paid, would be worked out between the health department, University Hospital, and the medical school.

The present nurseries would need to be completely rebuilt so that there would be a high-risk nursery constructed, and all equipment and personnel needed for this program would be paid for by the grant. It all pleased the local Health Department, but the County Health Officer said he would have to talk with Dr. Ira Myers, the State Public Health Officer, to get his permission to apply for the grant. I thought we might have an edge there, as Dr. Myers's daughter was one of our pediatric residents. She would later be killed in a raid on a church-sponsored hospital by the Taliban in Afghanistan in the first few weeks following the tragedy of September 11, 2001. She was serving as a missionary physician, taking care of Afghanistan women and children. Being a medical missionary was all she ever wanted to do.

After about a week we got a reply from Dr. Myers, who said he had no objection to our applying for the grant, but he could not allow just one county to apply. In order to prevent the perception that Jefferson county was being shown favoritism, at least one other county would need to apply along with us. If we could get a total of at least two Alabama counties to apply, it was all right.

This didn't seem insurmountable to me. It had to be a county that had somewhat the same facilities as Jefferson county, including a hospital that could build and staff a neonatal intensive care nursery. The only one that I could think of was Mobile county, with its county-owned hospital, Mobile General. I called Dr. Dan Sullivan, who practiced pediatrics in Mobile, and told him about the possible adolescent pregnancy program, the possibility for improving the teaching program for the pediatric residency program, and a neonatal intensive care nursery for Mobile county. He was excited about the possibilities and set up a meeting between himself, the county health officer, and me. I drove down, spent the night with my folks, and we had the meeting the next day. I don't remember the name of the county health officer, but I do remember that he had a definite British accent. I explained the whole deal as it should work, substituting Mobile General for University Hospital. I told him that I would write his grant application and all he would have to do was fill in the details as they applied to Mobile County. It was an "offer he couldn't refuse," and he didn't.

Now I had to get the financial details all smoothed out with the university. I made an appointment with Dr. Paul Brann, who was the medical center chief financial officer. He was an absolute genius at working out financial snags. I took over the grant request for him to look at, and I left him to look over my financial machinations. I got a call from him a little later saying that everything looked all right to him, except that we had one problem. The University of Alabama had never borrowed money in the history of the school. I said, "Well, it's time they did and joined the rest of us." He chuckled and said he would give it a try. In about a week he called me and, in an astonished tone of voice, declared that the trustees had agreed to our borrowing the money, since we had a guaranteed way to pay off the loan. So we had another first, though I don't know how distinguished it was. We got the University of Alabama to borrow money for the first time in its long, distinguished history.

Now I had to find me a neonatologist, since I had just applied for a grant that required one. I asked Russell Cunningham, who was on board now, if he knew any neonatology fellows up at Harvard that we might look at. He said that there was a very brilliant fellow over at Boston Lying-In Hospital who was finishing up his fellowship, but he thought that he had already accepted a position at the University of Virginia. The new chairman there was Bill Thurmond, the same fellow who was at Tulane when I came back south, and who had occupied the position I looked at with Tulane. The academic world in those days was very small. I was hard to discourage in those days, so I wrote this fellow, Dr. George Cassady, a letter asking him to visit us to look at what we were trying to build.

I received a letter in return saying that he was planning to join the University of Virginia, but he was going to the spring meetings in Seattle, Washington. He was going to present a paper on the use of oxygen electrodes to monitor premature infants. He suggested that maybe we could get together up there and talk over a drink. That didn't sound like he was just dying to join us. I hadn't planned on going to the spring meetings that year, since Seattle was such a long way away, but now it seemed that I was going. I asked my secretary to get me a flight and make hotel reservations, and I was off to the misty Northwest.

I checked into the hotel, ran into some of my old Minnesota buddies and then started looking for George. I finally went to the presentation of his paper, and I was impressed very much with his work. I sought him out after his talk, and we decided that we would have that drink and discuss things right then. We found a little bar around the corner from the hotel and sat and talked for awhile. I had my spiel down pat by now, and I added a little more about our role in making medicine available to everyone and the responsibility of a department to the state that makes everything possible. After thirty or forty minutes of my blabbering on about my dream for the department, he said, "I am going to visit my folks in Los Angeles, and I plan on leaving there on such and such a date. Why don't I just swing by Birmingham and visit with you on my way back to Boston?" I agreed with that and got a flight back home.

I never could get George to tell me what flight he was taking into Birmingham from Los Angeles, but I knew what day he was flying in. There weren't that many flights he could be on in those days, so I figured out which flight he had to be flying. I met his plane, and I could see the surprise on his face when he saw me. I took him to the hotel in the medical center, where we had made reservations for him, and took him out to dinner that night. We had steaks at Dale's Cellar, a local restaurant that was really located in a celler and had lots of atmosphere and good food. The next day we went to the fifth floor of the Hillman Building, where the entire floor had been gutted in preparation for building the high-risk nursery. The best talking job I ever did was talking the head of obstetrics into letting me have his old labor and delivery area as part of the high-risk nursery, where

I had spent a month being sleep-deprived and delivering babies.

The nursery had not been designed at that time, and I explained to George that whoever took this position was going to be able to design the nursery as he wanted. Then I showed him the space that had been reserved for the neonatal research lab area. The rest of the day was spent with him going around and talking with the dean, faculty members, and Harry Shirkey. By now, Harry had given up on having a residency at Children's. He also talked with the two lady members, who essentially had given up on overt opposition by now. They had pretty well given up on running the neonatal service by now, especially since I had gutted the Hillman nursery area. The next day we again went upstairs to the fifth floor, and I left him there to just look the area over at his leisure. After a bit, Hugh stuck his head into my office, and said, "Herschel, I think you've got him."

I replied, "Is that so? Why do you think that?"

Hugh grinned and said softly, "He's upstairs stepping off his lab area." Needless to say, George joined us, and Bill Thurmond didn't speak to me for months for stealing his neonatologist.

We and Mobile County both received the grants, and they are still in effect today. Pregnant adolescents are taken care of free of charge during their term, their delivery, and for a year afterward. Their babies are also cared for after delivery, and any hospital care needed for illness, or as the result of a premature birth for the same year. Formula is also provided during that postpartum year. This program is called the WIC program, and now it's obvious the reason why no other counties in Alabama have this to offer.

We now began having a pediatric resident rotate over to Children's Hospital, but in limited numbers. Harry was given an appointment as associate professor of pediatrics and was put in charge of the residency program when our residents rotated over there. Harry began working on a book in pediatric pharmacology that was edited by him with a large number of contributing authors. He worked very hard on this and other aspects of pediatric drugs, and he coined the term "pharmacologic orphans," referring to the lack of drugs available for children younger than six years of age. He became busy enough that we recruited a pediatrician from the FDA to help him. This was a cheerful guy who always seemed in a terrific upbeat mood. He had his training at the University of Cincinnati, which was where Harry probably first met him. Dr. Paul Palmisano was such an energetic and cheerful guy that it was almost impossible not to like him. I didn't know whether to list this field of pediatric pharmacology as a true subspecialist area or not. Although we listed this division along with the other subspecialty divisions, I must admit I never could accept it as one. It seemed to have only one aim, to get Harry's book published.

By the time that George got down to Alabama, the construction of the neonatal nursery was about finished. He had gotten it up and running, and we managed to get his lab all furnished. The equipment in George's research laboratory was not furnished by the nursery grant, nor did he have an NIH grant to purchase things needed for his research. It required a lot of talking with various sources, including pharmaceutical companies, and also some just plain begging before I was able to get that task accomplished.

It wasn't long before it became obvious that George was going to need some help. By now, our previous director of the nursery had left in a huff and had started working for the health department in well-baby clinics. We found a fellow up in Nashville at Vanderbilt School of Medicine who it seemed would fit in very nicely. Dr. Willard Blankenship joined us as assistant professor of pediatrics. It was getting easier to recruit people to join us now, as people were beginning to notice our growth and the quality of our people.

Charlie and Bill came back to rejoin us about this time. Bill didn't need a lab for his work, and we managed to get the funds to equip Charlie's virology laboratory. While at Harvard, he had worked mostly with the rubella (German measles) virus and its transfer across placental membranes to infect the baby. One afternoon, Jon Stromfjord, the director of the hospital laboratories, dropped in for a chat. He inquired, "What can you think of that we can routinely screen for in the newborns?" He said that he would love to set up routine screening programs for things that no one else screened for yet.

I replied, "Why don't you go down the hall and talk to Charlie Alford? He just got back from working on the rubella virus, its infection of the fetus, and the antibody response by the fetus. Perhaps you could set up a protein screening program on cord blood and be able to pick up fetal viral infections before they became clinically evident." Jon walked on down the hall and pretty soon he, Charlie, George, and Willard were engaged in an animated discussion that just brimmed with excitement. They found that the fetus does make antibodies against viruses such as rubella, herpes, etc. They published this work in the *New England Journal of Medicine*. They became overnight academic celebrities, and they continued this work for years. Charlie would eventually become national president of the Society of Pediatric Research. It was a long way from trying to measure the volume of bottles using an instrument whose data couldn't be replicated.

By now, the federal government was well involved in the day-to-day operation of the medical school. The hospitals and the new hospital buildings, dormitories, and classroom buildings sat on an area that had been swept clean through the auspices of the Department of Housing and Urban Development. This left the government feeling they had the right to oversee the programs that were located in those buildings that sat on the land they provided. All of the grants from NIH that were obtained through various faculty members carried overhead costs that had to be covered by the university. Dr. Volker laughed and told me one day, "One more grant and the university will go broke." He was laughing, but one could hear a tinge of truth in his voice.

At this same time, the state legislature began to put political pressure on Dr. Volker to stop allowing so much federal money into the running of the medical center. He told me, "The state supplies twenty percent of the medical center budget, and the federal government supplies about eighty percent. Who do they think I am going to listen to?"

It was about this time that the federal bureaucracy began to notice that there were fewer students going into the general practice of medicine than into the various medical and surgical specialties. By now, we had all learned that if a vacuum was in a program, the government was going to move in, and it did. The government's solution was to force physicians to go into general practice by vastly increasing the number of physicians graduating, thus filling up the need for specialists and causing physicians to go into general practice as a second resort. Obviously, they had never read C. Northcote Parkinson's *Book of Parkinson's Laws*. Parkinson's first law was that the work would always expand to take care of the people available. He developed this law while serving in the RAF during World War II. He was in charge of some clerical office, and the time came for the beginning of Christmas vacations. The staff started giving leaves to a few people at a time. As people left, the work was absorbed by the remaining crew and things began to seemingly work more efficiently. Finally, only he and one other man were left, with the work all done more quickly, and certainly more efficiently. This experience helped him form Parkinson's first law, "The work will expand to take care of the people available." Each chapter in his *Book of Parkinson's Laws* was a new law. These included how to tell who the important people at a cocktail party were or never to accept a job at an institution where they only bragged about one thing, how good the cafeteria food was, at the place.

True to Parkinson's first law, the result of this intervention was there were more specialists, each doing a little less work and each seeing a smaller number of patients. Eventually, subspecialties would continue to blossom in the everyday milieu of medical and surgical specialties. We arrived at a point one hundred eighty degrees from what the unwise legislation intended to solve. The plethora of specialists had vastly increased, and the physicians in small towns remained the same. This need eventually started to be met by graduates of foreign medical schools, mostly from the Latin countries of the Caribbean, Central and South America, India, and Pakistan. This situation exists to this day. Probably the worst thing that occurred in this entire thing was that the federal government had extended another tentacle into medical education and the daily practice of medicine. It would seem that the situation was very much like the old tales of making a deal with the devil; one paid an awful price for what ultimately was little gained in dealing with the government.

In another of my nightly scannings of the blue sheet I came across an item describing a new program being offered by the Children's Bureau, another government entity. It described funds being made available to health departments, university medical programs, and some carefully selected hospitals to develop and run comprehensive health programs for children up to nineteen years of age. It required that the applying agency put up one fourth of the cost of the projected cost in cash, or in-kind services, etc. That was not a difficulty because we already took care of most of the county's indigent care children with money provided by Jefferson County indigent care funds. We could declare the money that was already provided to us for the care of indigent children as our matching money. Again, I sent a short note to the dean and he answered, "Go for it."

Children's Bureau main offices for our area of the country were located in Atlanta. I soon became very familiar with the trip to and from Atlanta, the Children's Bureaum and its staff. We put together a program that involved public health and its well-baby clinics, the dental school's department of pediatric dentistry, Children's Hospital, University Hospital, surgery, radiology and most of all, us. The Children's Hospital would serve as the outpatient clinic, and children would be admitted there and the University Hospital. Pediatric dental clinics and Children's Hospital clinics in the county would be expanded and completely refurbished by the grant. Any equipment needed for the care of these children would be purchased and installed. The salaries for all types of physicians, nurses, and technicians were also included.

When we got it all planned and estimated the costs, it added up to 1.7 million annually, and we would be required to have our matching funds of slightly more than half a million. This amount of money was already being spent by the county and Community Chest funds at Children's Hospital. Now we simply used this money as our matching funds. Everyone that I showed it to said that I had bitten off more than I could possibly chew and I should scale it back. My reply was that we were already doing it; now we were just going to get paid for it. The worst that could happen was that we would be told, "No." Of course, my retort was all bravado, because in today's dollar value that would be about 17 million per year.

We submitted it, and to everyone's surprise we got the grant. This gave us money for recruiting and funding of more pediatric faculty, which we did as we could find them. The best thing was that now all the children that we cared for received the same level of care, and it was all funded either through private insurance or the grant. Dr. Sid Finn was so appreciative of what I got for the pediatric dental department that he made me a professor of pediatric dentistry.

I told him, "Sid, I don't know anything about pediatric dentistry."

He said, "Don't you worry; no one is going to ask you any questions."

As all this was transpiring, Dr. Champ Lyons, professor of surgery, developed a malignant brain tumor, and in a very short while he died. Now the medical school was faced with the job of finding a new chief of surgery. There had never been anyone else in that position but Dr. Lyons. I was one of the faculty members who were appointed to the search committee. We met and decided that we would send out letters to all the medical schools and request that they send us recommendations for surgical physicians whom they thought might make a good candidate. We took the candidates' names that were suggested and began to rank them according to our opinion of their desirability for the vacancy. Essentially, all the responders said that Dr. John Kirklin was the top man in the country, but no one thought he would leave his present position at the Mayo Clinic in Minnesota.

We had one or two candidates visit, but so far no one impressed us all that much. In one of our meetings Dr. Joe Reeves, the search committee chairman, broached the subject of asking Dr. Kirklin down. Joe expressed the thought that, just out of courtesy, perhaps we should extend an invitation. Joe knew him personally, and he said he would be glad to call and see how he reacted. John replied that he would be glad to come, but the schedule he offered for the visit did not indicate an overwhelming interest. He was going to fly down on Friday afternoon, spend the night, and fly back home late Saturday afternoon.

Well, he came and spent Friday evening talking with Dr. Harrison. Since he was a renowned cardiac surgeon it seemed a good way to start, since he and Dr. Harrison were well acquainted. Each of us met separately with him on Saturday morning, and we clinical types talked about our plans for our individual departments and where we were trying to take them. That afternoon he was shown around the hospital and medical center. He caught his plane, and we started to look at our candidate list again. About a week later, each member of the search committee received a large manila envelope about two inches thick. There was an enclosed letter stating that the University of Alabama Medical Center was very exciting to him. The enclosed papers were things that would have to be planned for the future if he were to come. We immediately met again and agreed to his terms.

They mainly dealt with things that needed to be done in the hospital to meet his requirements. His patients were usually very famous people, and we needed to have first-class accommodations to care for them. For instance, an Arab prince would come in and would want the entire floor for himself. The cost of this wasn't an issue for them.

When John finally moved down and assumed the chairmanship of the department of surgery, I was able to offer him a salary for a pediatric surgeon funded from our grant. He took my money very graciously and immediately hired the man second in command at

Boston Children's Hospital (Harvard) and established him at our Children's Hospital. We were in high cotton now.

I got a call one day from the dean telling me that the school wanted to nominate George Cassady for that year's Markle Scholarship. Every year, the Markle Foundation would select a young and upcoming faculty member from some university and present him with a financial award of thirty thousand dollars a year for five years to help his research work. The Administration chose George to be that year's candidate. The Dean wanted me to provide the documentation of George's life up to that moment. Now George was a very private person, and it was going to be difficult to obtain much private information from him. However, for the chance to be a Markle Scholar, he opened up some.

George had been a sickly child, being bedeviled by chronic asthma and innumerable allergies. He grew up in the Los Angeles area, and by then it was beginning to show the early signs of smog. He was homeschooled for the simple reason that when he went to school he was constantly sick. He began to play the piano, and because he had a lot of free time on his hands, he spent the majority of his time practicing the piano. He apparently became very good at it, and when he was twelve years old he was entered in a contest, the winner to be featured with the Los Angeles Symphony in a concert at the Hollywood Bowl. George won, and the boy he beat out was named Andre Previn. Mr. Previn became a world-renowned concert pianist, conductor of The Royal Philharmonic Orchestra of London, and held innumerable other honors. That win by George at the age of twelve was very impressive to me.

One night Nancy and I, along with George and his wife, were dinner guests of Willard Blankenship and his wife. After dinner the conversation somehow turned to pianists, and George made the comment that he could always tell the identity of a pianist by the way he pedaled. Willard said, "I find that hard to believe. I've got records by several pianists; I'm going to play them, and you tell me who they are." He played them, and George would identify them after only a few bars. That was truly an amazing performance. George didn't get the Markle Scholarship, but he was very heartened by the administration thinking highly enough of him to nominate him as their candidate.

Soon after we got the big grant from Children's Bureau, I got a call from Bill Daniels down in Montgomery. If you remember, I told you to remember his name when Hugh Dillon left Montgomery. He was the second person in what had been a three-man group before Hugh's departure.

He said, "When are you going to start an adolescent program up there?"

I immediately retorted, "Whenever you come up here to run it."

He replied, "O.K., I'll be up to talk with you about it."

And, he did. We set up a program strictly limited to care for adolescent children. We were able to fund it through our large grant from Children's Bureau. Bill was an extremely valuable addition to our department. He was big in the state medical society and the AMA. One can always use political connections.

Bill also was an absolutely tireless worker. He set up a clinic for teenagers, constantly wrote articles on their care, and eventually edited a book titled, *Adolescent Medicine*. It was an excellent book, very practical, and it sold like hotcakes. It was the first book of its kind in adolescent care. Bill eventually became president of the Adolescent Medicine Society. He was a marvel and an absolute pleasure to be around. He owned a Porsche roadster in which he spun around town. It was painted a bright, burnt-orange color, and his kids called it "The Pumpkin." I am sure that the people in Montgomery missed him as much as we enjoyed having him. I always felt a little guilty for stealing two members of that earlier three-man group. The poor fellow who was left with a solo practice never seemed to hold it against me. After Bill arrived, I found out something about him which I wasn't aware. He was the head of the pediatric medical service on the *Ship Hope*.

The *Ship Hope* was the brainchild of Robert Hope of Washington, D.C. He acquired an old hospital ship of World War II vintage and started a medical missionary program, which was totally different from anything tried before. He staffed the ship as a floating hospital, and they would dock in some country that had very rudimentary medical care.

The ship had a different mission than various programs offered by other organizations. They weren't there just to care for the sick, although they did plenty of it, but their mission was one of education of the medical community who were already there. They not only worked with physicians, but nurses, lab techs, various clinical staffing positions, and finally they set up a public health program. It was not unusual to have patients with tetanus, diphtheria, polio, etc. because there were no immunization programs in effect in most places they went.

The ship would stay for one year, and by departure time they had educated the locals so they could handle the programs from then on. They usually left two or three people in public health behind after that initial year because the programs for safe drinking water, sewage, and continuing the immunization programs would take longer to establish and maintain. The primary staff of the ship, such as nurses, technicians, administrative personnel, and the medical supervising physicians, would sign on for a year. The various medical specialty physicians would sign on for two-month rotations. Many of them were repeat volunteers who got great pleasure out of the work. Bill was in charge of getting the pediatricians signed on and the rosters filled. It was a great honor to be called a "Hopie." There is no *Ship Hope* anymore; the old boat's hull finally rusted out and was no longer seaworthy.

Bill got it in his head that I needed to go on the ship for a two-week tour as the first visiting professor on the ship. After some time of my trying to ignore him, I decided that I would go. He was not an easy man to ignore. The ship had just docked at Cartagena, Columbia, and I would fly down with a group of physicians starting their tour of two months. We deplaned and were picked up by vans belonging to the Hope project. There were two pediatricians, not including me. The ship had been changed very little from its tour of duty in World War II. We physicians slept in one large room, with access to a deck located on the side of the ship. A lot of the fellows took advantage of this to get their tans intensified. You have to remember that this was before anyone had made the connection of sun exposure and melanoma.

The big room was filled with row upon row of double-decked bunks, which were probably part of the original equipment. We didn't spend much time there anyway, as almost every minute was utilized. We awoke, usually showered, and made our way down to the mess hall. They prepared anything that anyone could possibly want; what impressed me most was the supply of tropical fruits. All kinds of bananas, pineapple, mango, etc., were all served in abundance, and I am sure they were all picked fresh the day before.

Everyone wore white clothing, and we were all issued a little round pin slightly smaller than a dime. It was inscribed with the name *Ship Hope* on it. That way, any of the locals would know we were associated with the ship. The first morning, they took us to the local hospital where we would be working every day. It was an absolutely beautiful white stucco building with red-tiled roofs in the classic style of Spanish architecture. The building was built in the shape of a two-story "U," with balconies on the second floor exhibiting enormous red-flowered bougainvillea surrounding a green lawn in the patio below. The building had been built in the 1500s, and not a lot done to it since then.

We went into the pediatric ward, which had small iron beds aligned perpendicular to the walls. I couldn't tell whether the floor was dirt or concrete, but later determined it was made of flat stones. The iron beds were fitted with bare, coiled springs about three-inches thick which were covered by dirty cotton mattresses about three inches thick. The beds certainly didn't look to be the most comfortable beds in the world, but I am sure that they easily surpassed anything that these children had at home—if they had a physical structure for a home. Over in one corner of the room we could see a large, conical mound of something about four- or five-feet tall. As we approached this mass, it became obvious that it was sweepings from the floor that had been painstakingly swept into that particular corner for decades, if not centuries. Later we found that the sterilizer for the operating room had been broken for the past two weeks, but it had not deterred the surgeons from operating. I really don't know what their infectious rate post-op was.

The hospital was surrounded by a large brick whitewashed wall that was about two-feet thick and ten- or twelve-feet high. It had one set of double gates which were enormous wrought-iron structures that took a good-sized man to open or close them. Every day at 5:00 p.m. those gates were closed, no matter how many people were waiting for care. Running in front of the hospital was a narrow street that barely allowed a single car to drive one way if there were no parking. On the corner stood a shop that sold caskets, and they showed their wares by standing the caskets on end and leaning them against the side wall, where they spanned the sidewalk and they actually protruded a little into the narrow street. There were all kinds of caskets displayed, from mahogany ones to ones made from Styrofoam.

They then took us to the pediatric clinic, which was located in an open-aired space on a large veranda. We began to see patients, and that is when one of the pediatricians pulled out an implement from his bag. This was not his first tour on the *Hope*, and he said that he learned from his earlier experiences on the *Hope* that this tool was definitely needed. With that, he pulled out a flyswatter. You could watch him on his clinic-duty days, and see him happily smashing away at those pesky critters. In the middle of the morning, they served us pure Colombian coffee. There was one thing that I became acutely aware of, they don't ship their good Colombian coffee to the United States. This coffee was black as India ink, but was sweet, delicately flavored, and the most delicious coffee without cream or sugar that I ever drank before or after that time. I have bought every brand of pure Colombian sold in America and it confirms my suspicions: we get only what they don't want up here in North America.

That afternoon, they showed me a problem they were having with a small round building located in the patio area. This building was not built at the same time as the main hospital; it was much younger and not nearly as pretty. It was perfectly round, with only one door. Inside the room was dimly lit and completely devoid of any furnishings. There was a small room about the size of a large closet to one side, and it contained the nurses' desk and shelves for holding supplies. Around the wall was a bare shelf about waist-high and about three-feet wide. There were IV hooks mounted on the walls about every two or three feet. The infants who were admitted to this house all had diarrhea and required IV fluids. They were placed on the shelf and given intravenous fluids. I don't know what their mortality rate was from the diarrhea and vomiting, but I would guess that it was high. I don't think they had the equipment for measuring serum electrolytes in micro quantities.

They were having a much more dire problem, however. Almost every child who was admitted to that unit was dying of pseudomonas septicemia. That is, every child who was admitted to the unit developed a bloodstream infection with a very wicked germ named pseudomonas, and they essentially all died. Since this was a hospital-derived infection, the only solution to this was to shut the unit down. Then they needed to get in some fresh air by opening the door and tiny windows, throwing everything out (since there were no furnishings), and burning anything that might be harboring the germ. It took about a week to convince them to do this. The unit was shut down, cleaned, and scrubbed with lots of soap, and when they moved back in after a few days there was no recurrence.

There was no middle class in Columbia. The citizens were either rich, with all the amenities that brings, or one was pitifully poor. There is no life insurance available for the poor, so they look upon their children as their old-age caretakers. The infant mortality was around fifty percent when I was there, so the poor had to have a lot of children to insure there being someone to care for them in their old age. Death of a child was an expected thing, and the parents just grew to accept it as a way of life. When we were having all the deaths of infants, I had the opportunity to be around when parents were told that their child had died. There was absolutely no emotion demonstrated by either parent.

They would gather their family around them and accept the child's body, which would be wrapped in some type of material. They would then walk across the street to the casket shop, in some way purchase a small casket made of Styrofoam, and place the body in it. The father would place the pure white casket on his head and start walking to the cemetery, which was three or four blocks away. The mother, other children, and any other family members would follow in single file as they began the trek to bury their child. There was nothing like embalming, wakes, and such things that we are so fond of in the United States. In the whole process there would not be a tear shed, only immobile faces staring straight ahead. I suppose that the father would dig the grave, place the tiny casket into it, and cover it with dirt. I doubt that the grave would be marked, except perhaps by some wooden marker as simple as a stake.

Fortunately, the *Ship Hope* furnished me a full-time interpreter. It was a good thing, because my Spanish was limited to "*si-si*" and "*adios*." My interpreter was a young, black-headed girl with white skin, which meant that she was one of the elite. She spoke excellent English with hardly any accent. She was married but I never met her husband, and I presumed they had no children. She would be at the ship every morning and would stay with me until things began to slow down around five o'clock. We rode in one of the *Hope* vans, which would chauffeur us around wherever we wanted to go.

In this manner, I got to see a lot of the city that I would not have seen otherwise. The utter poverty was ghastly. A large percentage of the population had no housing but would use all sorts of methods to identify a small bit of space to which they claimed temporary custody. Walking out into an open grassy area, they would take small tree branches and stick them into the earth to delineate a small square of land that would be called their home. There would be no privacy because the branches were never close enough together to even suggest they were trying to accomplish that. It was just a way to state to the world, *This is my place, and I and my family live here*.

I spent my time most days making rounds with the local pediatricians, teaching, lecturing, and helping the lab techs with their hematological preparations. One day, a pediatrician from the medical school in Bogota appeared during some of the teaching sessions. He asked me if I would come speak to the students and pediatric faculty at National University on my way back to the United States. I told him that I would be honored.

One day I rode with one of the public health teams that was going out to an outlying village to immunize essentially all of the people in that small village. We arrived and drove into the center of town, which consisted mostly of wooden or grass shacks arranged around a common area completely void of foliage. Naked children were scooting around in all directions, and when it became time to immunize them, the parents started shooing them all into one location. It reminded me of chickens being herded into one area when I was a boy. I was amazed at the efficiency with which it all was carried out.

My time on the *Hope* drew to a close, and I had enjoyed it immensely. I was driven out to the airport, said good-bye to everyone, and took off for the capital. Bogota is built in the mountains, and when I first arrived I would tire very easily, but I became acclimated in just a short time. I spent my first day just walking around and seeing the city. Since Columbia is one of the main centers for emeralds, I spent part of my time shopping for one for Nancy. I made a bad purchase, as the jewelry piece that I selected was too primitive. However, it did have a nice stone, and I have been told that it is the thought that counts.

The next day, representatives from the university picked me up and we drove out to the University Hospital. I gave my little talk on anemia, and they presented some patients for discussion. After it was over a short, thin man approached me and said, "Dr. Bentley, I am on the pediatric faculty here, but I wondered if you might have an opening for someone to come to your school and train in neonatology?" Just like that, George and the department had its first fellow. One never knows when the good things are going to happen.

When I got back home, I began to think of things that would

enhance the depth of the department, improve our image so as to attract high-performing pediatric residency positions, and set us somewhat apart from the run-of-the-mill pediatric departments. I began to allow myself the luxury of really dreaming big dreams. Slowly the thoughts of getting someone to endow a chair in pediatrics started creeping into my thoughts. There was not an endowed chair in the University of Alabama Medical Center. I really didn't know if one existed on the main campus or not. I started to find what was required to have an endowed chair. The best of all worlds at that time was for someone to make a donation of 1 million dollars as an endowment to support the individual who was named for the spot. Since that time, I am sure the cost of endowing a chair has probably risen tenfold. Of course, the number of people likely to have that sort of money has risen equally. The idea is that the money is invested, and the professor's salary is derived from the earnings, never from the principal.

Try as I might, I just couldn't come up with any names of individuals who were that engrossed in the care of children and who might have 1 million dollars to give away. Things were beginning to look bleak for my desired endowed chair. Then I began to think of getting a foundation to endow a chair. After all, foundations are created to give away money to causes to which they are devoted. Somehow I became aware of the Meyer Foundation located in Birmingham. They periodically had given money to Children's Hospital, so they must have had some interest in sick children.

I made contact with them through the simple act of looking up the foundation's name in the phone book and calling the director. He wasn't too enthusiastic about the idea, but he said he would bring up the subject to his board of directors at a future meeting. Well, I figured that was not the way someone who was overly enthused over the proposal would act, but they hadn't said "no" yet. However, I had been turned down by enough people to whom I had presented my dreams that I thought I had recognized a polite brush-off. There was at that time a book published with all the foundations in the United States listed, with detailed descriptions of the foundation's interests, amount of money awarded in the past, etc.

I had resorted to leafing through this book when I received a call from a Mr. Bill Rushton. I recognized the name. His father was president of the Protective Life Insurance Co. when Nancy worked there in the actuarial department, and she called his son Billy.

I answered the call and found that he was calling for the Meyer Foundation. It seemed that the board of directors was intrigued by the idea and wanted to discuss it further. Bill was very polite, earnest and friendly. He remembered Nancy, and we immediately got along very well. It would turn out that he would lead me through the entire trail that we had to follow to make our endowed chair a reality.

They were hesitant about giving us a lump sum of money, but were receptive to the idea of their keeping the principal but providing the money earned from investments on a million dollars on a yearly basis. After many meetings with Dr. Paul Brann, the school's money man, and Bill Rushton, this plan was adopted, and we had a funded chair entitled The Meyer Research Professor of Pediatrics. Now we had to find someone to put in it. We wanted to recruit someone who was young enough to be around for a while, who was established in the research world, and whose name was familiar enough that we would attract some positive publicity for the appointment.

We started looking, and we had several good candidates to come down. Some were interested in the position and some weren't. The problem was that we hadn't talked to anyone in whom I was particularly interested. Suddenly, it occurred to me that we had interviewed no one who was better than, or even the equal of, Charlie Alford. I got approval from the dean, and I asked Charlie to drop by the office. I said, "Charlie, we have decided to offer you the research chair appointment."

Charlie answered, "Will you get into any trouble offering me this?" This was several years before his election as president of The Society of Pediatric Research, so I guess my choice was vindicated in full.

We now had added Dr. Max Cooper from Bob Good's bailiwick in Minnesota. It was his job to get us up to speed in immunology. Also, we had hired Dr. Josh Carey as associate professor of pediatric Neurology. Josh was a rotund little man who was truly jolly. He also had a PhD in neuroanatomy, and he had been collaborating with neuroanatomists down the hall for several years. This was a group working on the evolution of the central nervous system. Josh's experimental animal was the turtle, because almost all of its brain was devoted to the sole function of locomotion. Josh could usually be identified from a distance because he always wore wide, bright-red suspenders. He had a deep resonant voice, and his deep, throaty belly laugh would put Santa Claus to shame. He loved to have people to his home for breakfast, where he would serve sourdough flapjacks. In his backyard was a large wire-enclosed pen, and as would be expected, it was completely filled with different species of turtles.

Around this time, I was invited to the Columbus, Georgia, hospital to conduct teaching rounds with their house staff. I drove down and spent most of the day talking and going on rounds, and I drove back home that afternoon. A few days later I received a call from Dr. Ralph Tiller in Columbus. He told me that he wanted to come to Birmingham to discuss the possibility of being a part of our teaching program. He had a private practice in Columbus and was very involved in the pediatric residency program. His wife, Mary, was also a physician and worked for the public health department. He drove up, accompanied by his wife. I had alerted the public health officer of her coming up and that she might be looking for a job. With all the money I had gotten them by way of grants, they were more than willing to cooperate.

Ralph went around talking to the members of the pediatric department and the administration. I had been doing a little investigation, and everyone who was connected with him in any way was deeply impressed, not only by his depth of general pediatric knowledge but also by his integrity. I found that he was very interested in pulmonary disease and wanted to get some further training. I made him an offer he couldn't refuse. I wanted him to take charge of the pediatric outpatient program and get it straightened out. I had always wanted to get someone with outpatient experience to take over that role in our teaching program. With the added patient load resulting from the big grant, it had just overwhelmed our female director.

I must admit that when I informed her that she was being demoted to one of the teacher positions in the clinic, she wasn't overjoyed by the news. She had always considered the outpatient area to be her sole possession, so it did take a little time for her to become accustomed to the idea. Ralph took over the cystic fibrosis clinic, which was a relief to me, since I was the soul physician in that particular clinic. In a relatively short time, the outpatient program was well organized and functioning smoothly. Ralph and I went duck hunting a lot down in Fairhope, Alabama, on a friend's farm, and Hugh, Ralph, and I went quail hunting frequently on his old hunting grounds around Columbus, Georgia. Life was getting to be better. Ralph continued to want further pulmonary training, and he arranged to do this at Tulane University, so we had a pulmonary disease sub-specialist.

I was maintaining a fairly active hematology and oncology service. Referrals had increased a great deal since the initial months. One day a physician from Union Springs, Alabama, came to see me with one of his adopted, identical golden-haired twin girls. She was found to have acute lymphatic leukemia, and we were very concerned that her identical twin might develop the same problem. For some reason, as it seems to occur in physician's children more frequently than chance, treatment did not go well. We were never able to get her into a smooth remission. She had an awful lot of complications, and I often needed help from the pediatric surgeon, Dr. Marshall Pitts, and my old buddy Hugh.

The child died about six months after beginning chemotherapy. The night that she died, her father and I were walking through the bowels of the hospital to sign papers connected with the death, release of the body, etc., and I said, "I am very sorry that we just weren't able to really help her much."

He replied, "Don't worry, Herschel, I did all my grieving six months ago." His other twin did not develop leukemia. However, his adopted son was playing with a propeller-driven small rocket, and as he released his hold on the rocket it rose rapidly and the propeller slashed his right eyeball. He permanently lost sight in that eye. About three years later, the physician himself dropped dead of a coronary occlusion. I have often thought about the amount of grief that the mother suffered in such a short time and so early in her life. She was a lovely, gracious young Jewish mother.

Around two months after the death of his daughter, the father called me and said that he wanted to do something for the physicians who helped take care of his daughter, since none of us charged him as a matter of professional courtesy. In order to understand his gift to us, a person must understand Union Springs, Alabama. Union Springs is located in the Black Belt of Alabama, so named for the color of the soil. The area around is rolling low hills covered with grasslands and pine forests. In this area, many of the old, rich families of America and their companies have bought thousands of acres of the land around Union Springs. They have given the plantations their names, such as Maytag Plantation and Du Pont Plantation.

The only thing they are raised on is wild quail. They plant strips of quail food such as chick peas, etc., and make sure that adequate water is available. The plantation is run full time by hired on-site caretakers who insure the quail do well and that no one hunts there illegally. The supervisor of Maytag Plantation was a patient of our patient's father, and through him he had made arrangements for us to have a day's hunt on the plantation. We drove down the day before the hunt and stayed at the home of our hosts. They gave a very nice dinner party in our honor with local people present.

The next morning we awoke with a feeling of great expectation and enthusiasm. We received our directions as to how to get to the plantation and off we went. We turned off the narrow country highway onto a long curved drive. As we topped a hill, there lay this enormous one-story plantation home. It must have been one hundred and fifty feet in width with a railed front porch that stretched the entire width of the house. The front porch was filled with high-backed rocking chairs as a place of rest and recreation for the Maytags' regular guests. We had previously been told to circle the house and come around to the back. When we did, there before us was a sight I am sure rivaled the olden days of big hunts. There were big bonfires going, horses, wagons containing dog cages filled with field champion dogs, and riders to meet our needs for the hunt. Hugh turned to me and said excitedly, "Boy, Herschel, we are going to live like white folks today."

Each of us was given a horse to ride. Mine was a small, gray horse whose name was Castro. He was so named because Castro had ridden him in a parade in New York City when he visited the United Nations. Luckily he was very gentle because I had not ridden a horse since my boyhood in Amory. The manager of the hunt was the supervisor of the plantation. He was surprisingly young and very cordial. He made us feel as if we belonged there. There were certain rules that we had to follow. We only shot on covey rises, and we were not allowed to shoot any singles that we might walk up after the quail covey lifted off. We had a quail limit, but I don't recall what it was. It followed whatever guidelines the state issued that year. When the dogs pointed a covey, two of us would get off the horses and approach the pointed covey until the birds flushed. No one else would get off the horses.

After the indoctrination, three dogs were released from the cages on the wagons. They were all field champion dogs, and there must have a total of fifteen of them. The dogs were told to hunt and immediately they began running and sniffing. The outriders began to fan out ahead of us, and in just a very few minutes the dogs were out of sight. They were long rangers, and we needed those outriders to keep them in sight. In a short time, one of the outriders stood up in his stirrups, waved his hat high in the air, and let out a high pitched "Yahoo!" We quickly rode over where one dog was on point and the two others were backing him up. Hugh and I got off and walked the birds up.

There must have been forty or fifty birds in that first covey. They were so thick that it would have been hard to miss if he had only shot amongst them. Hugh and I shot two birds each on that initial rise, and suddenly we began to calculate that we would reach the bird limit in about thirty minutes if we continued at that rate. We decided to shoot only one bird on a rise unless we accidentally shot two by mistake. On the next rise, Hugh and Marshall shot. Marshall had never been bird hunting before, and he quickly proved that a hunter could truly miss all the birds if he just shot amongst them. After that, Hugh and I would shoot one in front of him and one in front of us.

In about an hour, we came upon a small glen where another bonfire blazed and there was hot coffee and some refreshments. No strong drinks were present, as alcohol is a definite no-no on a hunt. They put up our dogs and brought out three more field champions, and we were off again. By the end of the morning we had our limit, despite our attempts to keep our numbers low on each covey rise. Never before, and never since, have I had such an experience. I realized that I could get accustomed to that in a hurry if it were available to me. Oh well, dream on.

Again back at the medical center, during one of my nightly perusals through the blue page report I came across an item that the federal government was going to construct six buildings at various universities yet to be chosen. These would be devoted to provide laboratory space for individuals in any science that touched upon the causes, cures, and management of mentally retarded individuals. In addition, there would be fifteen buildings built that would develop the practical applications to teach the teachers of retarded individuals according to the individual etiology of their mental retardation. In addition, specific teaching material would be developed that was tailored to the etiologies of specific mental deficiencies. The future teachers could then be taught how to best teach the individual students according to their specific deficiencies of central nervous system functions. The knowledge of how to determine and identify the specific deficiencies was to be the function of the six research programs.

It was a well-known fact that President Kennedy had a sister who was mentally retarded, and he was vitally interested in promoting development of programs that would delve into the various causes and possible prevention of such afflicted children. Dr. Robert Cooke, a boyhood friend of the Kennedys and also the current professor and chairman of pediatrics at John's Hopkins University, had two children with retardation. Again, I dictated a note to the dean. Likewise, again, I had a mandate to explore our applying for one of the grants by return memo. As I read the list of the different academic disciplines that were mandated to be included in this building, I then realized that all of them were expected to be meshed in some way, so that a basically unified educated product would be forthcoming.

I began to gather my thoughts about mentally retarded individuals. The condition causes most people to be very uneasy when mentally retarded individuals are around. Just like people tend to talk loudly around blind individuals, most individuals have an uneasy feeling around people with any type of serious disability. People rarely ever think of mentally retarded people as having diverse problems. In actuality, they are a conglomeration of many different causes, all being lumped under one banner: mental retardation. A person needs to go back to the old "experiments of nature" way of thinking. Physicians must approach them as individual patients with one of a conglomeration of central nervous system alterations that have an end result of something called mental retardation. Additionally, the medical community must learn to consider them as separate entities and not as a congealed mass. For instance, some of these conditions are not even identified yet, since we don't know how the abnormal varies from the normal because we don't know how the normal works.

What happens to a person's brain that causes it to be unable to store information? Some will be able to absorb knowledge to the level of a five-year-old, while others may be educated to the level of a seven-year-old. Then others will not rise above the level of an infant. The reason we can't fathom the differences between them is that we have very little information available as to how the brain stores knowledge and then recalls it for further use. Many etiologies we do know something about. Down's syndrome is a condition characterized by epicanthal folds of the eyelids which are wide spaced, small in-turned fifth fingers on both hands, different types of congenital heart disease, changes of the hips and arms, and mental retardation. Most of these, but not all of them, occur because of an abnormal chromosome.

Yet, as far as I know, no one has delved into exactly what alterations have occurred in the defective chromosome that causes these recurring parts of the syndrome. Then how do they differ from the children with the same findings that make up the syndrome but don't have a demonstrable alteration in that same chromosome? The findings of an abnormal chromosome, along with the changing of the name from Mongolian Idiocy to Down's syndrome, which makes it a less demeaning terminology, are about the only meaningful things that have occurred with this condition since I have been in medicine.

This problem must be approached in the same way that the physician did with his small patient who had repeated infections. First he must find what is normal before he can identify the abnormal. The aim for this money was to build these research and teaching institutes that were supposed to do just that.

I started to discover what individual departments were required to be included in this building and what their contributions were supposed to be. Then I found out that some of them, like special education, speech and hearing, sociology, and psychology didn't exist on our campus. Obviously they were going to have to create satellite programs from the main campus up to Birmingham. It seemed simple to me. That was before I went down to the main campus and found out that the sociology, speech, and hearing departments didn't speak to each other. What kind of nonsense was this? Grown men in charge of university departments were acting like teenagers and not speaking to each other! I solved it very diplomatically. I simply told them that there was going to be a lot of money available to each department with this grant, and if they wanted to share in it, they had better have mended their differences by the time I returned. I never realized that I had such tact.

I met with Dr. Joe Volker and with the dean, Dr. Dick Hill, about designing a building. Dr. Volker picked up the phone and called an architectural firm and informed them that we were going to apply for funds to construct a building in the medical center. He asked them if they would be interested in working with us in preparing working draft drawings, with no guarantee of payment if we didn't get the grant. The fellow said he would and suddenly, I was in the business of designing a six-story building. Dr. Volker then told me his theory of these kinds of dealings. He said, "Do you want a bank to be nice to you? Then you need to owe them lots of money. If you only owe them a small amount, they will harass you, but if you owe them a lot of money then they will be extremely nice because they don't want to make you mad."

I went over to the architect's office, and he started pulling plans of previous buildings he had designed and built out of drawers. In a short while, we had six floors with preliminary spaces and drawings and an outside building design. It was another box, like all the other new buildings on the campus. That was all that architects ever designed in those days.

After we got our grant prepared, I had to present it to the board of trustees and to the university president, Dr. Frank Rose. Before this was over, he knew my name. They approved it and we submitted the grant for the research building.

The government was only going to build six, but I thought we had a good chance of getting one.

I was wrong, we didn't get one. In the refusal, they reminded us of the fifteen buildings for teaching that were going to be awarded, and they encouraged us to apply. We did, and I sent the same grant back in. I got a call from the director of these projects and he said, "You have sent me the exact same grant that you submitted before."

I responded, "Yeah, I know. I plan to teach people how to do research."

He said, "OK." We got the grant.

Now, I had to find a way to come up with the money to pay for our matching funds for the grant. The government would give us four dollars for every one dollar of our own money. Since the Kennedy Foundation was so interested in mental retardation, I thought that it might want to give us the money to pay our matching funds. I made application, and we corresponded by letter and phone. Eventually the foundation sent down a committee that spent an entire day with us. The sociology chairman got up in the site committee meeting and claimed he wasn't sure what his role was supposed to be. I ignored him, and so did everyone else. I really felt sorry for him, as he made a complete ass out of himself. As Abe Lincoln said, "It is better to be quiet and be thought a fool than to open one's mouth and prove it." We didn't get the money from the Kennedy Foundation. Dr. Volker got the money from the Guy Sparks (a previous governor of the state) Foundation, and the building is so named.

While all of this was going on, the patient load on the pediatric floors at University Hospital had increased substantially and, in addition, the twelfth floor was being claimed for surgery expansion. That was going to rob us of our isolation unit. I talked with the hospital administration, and they agreed to renovate the entire fourth floor for pediatrics, which would include a new isolation unit. When they finished, they had done a remarkably good job. The pediatric floor was actually going to be pretty. Previously, it had all been colored that universal government green.

Now the university was faced with the knotty problem of how to integrate Children's Hospital with the University Pediatric Program, which included not only medicine, but also surgery, radiology, etc. Around the country, all such mergers are usually done with the chairman of pediatrics becoming the hospital director. Likewise, the head of surgery at Children's Hospital would be the head of the division of pediatric surgery in the department of surgery. This ties the Children's Hospital tightly to the teaching programs of the university. This created some problems within the ranks of the hospital practicing physicians. Some would lose their involvement in the day-to-day operation of overall patient care and the absolute autonomy of the private physicians in patient care if they were planning to avail themselves of house staff physicians and departmental personnel. In a teaching program, the quality of patient care would be under the scrutiny of the teaching staff. Everything would be held at a little higher standard, and this made everyone a little uneasy.

This made the issue of the chairman of the department of pediatrics being the hospital director a very thorny problem. The private physicians, particularly, didn't like this idea, and some even got the new Baptist Hospital to open a pediatric wing and began admitting their patients to this new unit. Prior to this time, there were no pediatric beds in the city except Children's and University Hospitals. The board of trustees of Children's did not want to fire Harry Shirkey for no reason, and they didn't want me moving in as hospital director. In their eyes it would seem as if they kicked Harry out to allow my moving in, because everyone was aware that the university was expecting this to occur.

As it was explained to me by Dean Hill, the solution that they worked out was that Harry would be removed as hospital director. He had been offered the same position at the Children's Hospital in Hawaii, so he would just accept the offer and go. I now became the problem, and their solution was to remove me from the chairmanship of pediatrics, but I would remain as professor of pediatrics. Since I had tenure they were not able to just let me go with a severance package if I elected to contest it. A new chairman would be appointed, and everyone would be happy. That solution I hadn't expected, and it took me a while to digest it. I felt like my staying would create a huge problem for the new chairman. I had recruited all thirty-four members of the faculty, mainly because we had all thought alike and had dreamed the same dream.

If I stayed, everyone would look at me to see what I thought whenever a decision was made. Eventually, that would lead to an untenable situation. Scotty McCallum came by to talk with me about it, and after hearing my thoughts on the matter, he agreed with me. He was the only person to express regret to me that I was leaving.

I tendered my resignation and, as I dropped it off at the dean's office, I began to ruminate on my tenure as chairman. When I took over, there were three people in the department. Of these three, two didn't particularly like the third too much. Now, there were thirty-four faculty members, all funded. When I was given my first budget, it totaled one hundred twenty-five thousand dollars a year; now it was 1.2 million, with a full-time accountant to keep it straight. I have a hard time with my private checkbook, so having a full-time accountant was a prudent thing. All of the sub-specialties in pediatrics except gastrointestinal services were now covered, and fellowships training in the other sub-specialty areas of the department were increasingly common. There had been two books published out of the department, and research papers flowed out in a steady stream. The indigent patients in Jefferson County and some in Mobile County were now given care at a high standard level, and it was all paid for. The pediatric services were now headquartered at Children's Hospital, and the quality of the staff was great. At that time, according to someone who does such things, the department was ranked fourth in the country. In addition, the hospitals, Children's University, other departments, as well as the public health department, were all beneficiaries of my grant labors. I didn't feel like I had done a bad job.

The day I left I went by the dean's office to say good-bye, but he was too busy to see me. I went up to the pediatric department, and there was literally no one there. I rolled my desk chair out (it was my private property) and put a few boxes of personal items in the seat. I went down on the back elevator, put my belongings in a U-Haul trailer, and I drove away. As I drove, a thought flitted through my brain—a person would think that, after working here for so long and so hard, he would have more things to take with him.

Bill Benton succeeded me as chairman, and after he retired from that position, Hugh Dillon took over until he died of multiple myeloma. Bill died during open heart surgery not too long after his retirement. Charlie died not too long ago while attending a social function. I am the sole survivor of the original crusaders.

I have been back only once since that day I drove away. That was to attend a gastrointestinal conference at Children's for continuing education credits. I didn't see anyone that I knew until, at a coffee break, Dr. Walter Cain approached me. Walter was a pediatric surgeon who had been around during all of our building days, and he was next on the program. He came up, shook my hand and said, "What do you think of all of this, Herschel? You built it." I mumbled something about it looking good, and after chatting a few minutes, he left to get ready for his teaching session.

I thought, "It's come a long way since we put on the first continuing education course ever given at the medical center." I turned back to the pediatric faculty members standing around the coffee urn who had been listening while the conversation had been going on and I explained, "I used to be chairman of pediatrics here." They nodded in acknowledgment and mumbled something in return, but just stared at me in a very strange way. Maybe they had previously thought that I was dead.

I have never been back since. A lot of the things I started, I never saw in operation, such as the mental retardation building, the fourth floor renovation with patients in it, etc. I feel fairly certain that the program in mental retardation was never assembled and working in a cohesive manner, tying etiology to teaching methods. The Regional Outpatient Program envisioned for the state certainly wasn't implemented. When the best brains in the legislature got through with it, it was solely a residential facility where families could rid themselves of the responsibility of trying to give the most education they could to their children. It was just what the state needed, another residential facility with nothing new being done.

The regional center built in Mobile is closed now, and essentially all the buildings have been sold.

Since then, I haven't been boycotting the place; I just have never been invited back. My mother always told me, "Never go where you're not wanted; it will only lead to trouble." I have followed her advice, in this matter anyway, all of my adult life.

Chapter 11

Arkansas Days — Changes are Not Always Wanted, Even the Good Ones

Now I was at a point in my life where I was going to do what I thought I was meant to do. I was going to set up a one-man practice in a small town and take good care of my private patients. I looked into going to Fairhope, Alabama, again. It seemed to me, with all the new influx of people in the area, it would be a good place to grow a private practice. I started looking for land to build an office, found a good lot that I could afford to buy, and ordered some office furniture. Fortunately, I didn't order much, just a couple of small couches. The lot was a nice one right on Greeno Road, and today it is right in the middle of a large new shopping center. It is worth a lot more now than it was then.

I was about two days short of closing on the land when I got a call from Ted Panos at the University of Arkansas School of Medicine in Little Rock, where he was professor and chairman of the department of pediatrics. Ted and I had become friends through our association at the pediatric chairmen meetings through the years. He said, "Herschel, I know you are having a lot of people call you now, but I was calling to see if you'd want to consider joining me up here and straightening out our outpatient clinic." He continued, "This thing has gotten to be such a mess that I need a strong person to put it in good shape."

I answered, "Well, in answer to your first statement, I haven't had any calls from other departments. Second, your call came at an opportune time, as I was about to settle on buying a lot here in Fairhope for a clinic of my own. However, if you are in a bind, I'll be happy to come out and see if I can find a way to help you out in a short time span." We settled on a time for me to come, and I canceled the meeting to close on the lot. I drove out to Little Rock, Arkansas, a few days later and got my first look at the Arkansas Medical Center.

Ted was such a pleasant and happy man that it was a pure pleasure to visit with him. After looking at the outpatient program, it was not hard to see what the problem was. Laziness was overwhelming. The woman who was running the outpatient unit had received good training; she was an old Minnesota program graduate. However, she had lost her zest for working and teaching, and the teaching program ran at a snail's pace. Another problem was that she was married to the head of surgery, which for some reason led her to think she could do as she chose. This was the main reason for the dwindling production of work, and Ted didn't want to cause friction between himself and the surgery program. The head of surgery was such a small enough person professionally that he would allow it to happen. Unfortunately, he was a very petty man.

Ted wanted me to handle this problem, just like I used Ralph Tiller to handle my outpatient problem. I figured that maybe I had this in my future as a way to serve my atonement for what I had asked of Ralph Tiller. I talked with Ted about his desires for the outpatient program and exactly what kind of program he wanted. Suddenly, that same calm that I had experienced when talking with Dean Hill about the chair at Alabama came over me, and I felt like this is what I am supposed to do. I accepted the position. I really didn't think that I would be there long, and I could get back to my own plans in about a year.

I found an apartment for us, and we moved our stuff in. After a short while we found a two-story red-brick house out close to the country club. Neither of us played golf, so the close vicinity to the country club wasn't all that big a draw. The yard needed a good bit of work, and I quickly found out why Little Rock got its name. The ground was literally filled with round, smooth rocks about six to eight inches in diameter. When trying to dig a small hole that would be the proper size for a small plant, there would be two to three round rocks and about one shovelful of dirt. I had to buy a truckload of top soil so I would have dirt to fill in the vacant space remaining in a hole where I had removed the rocks.

Landscaping the yard was very laborious toil that didn't allow any semblance of speed. Finally, one of the guys in the department gave me a steel pole about eight-feet long. It was pointed on one end and wedged shaped on the other, and it was perfect for wedging rocks out of potential holes. I found that just about everyone in the city had one of these steel poles, and they were standard merchandise in the hardware stores and garden shops.

I changed the design of the inner workings of the pediatric clinic so it began to function smoothly. Even the students began to comment on the improvement. Of course, I had alienated the former director by changing everything she had set up, but there was no other way to do it. However, at the same time that I alienated her, I found that I had done the same thing to her husband, the surgery chief. He considered himself too important to the Medical Center for anyone to allow this to happen. He took it to be a personal affront. Later this would be a problem for me, but now it was of little consequence. At least he was irked with me and not Ted.

This all was accomplished in about three months, and I began to realize that I was becoming bored with the dull routine of it.

I had experienced one really positive thing in my outpatient service: one of the medical students in the clinic was from Mountain Home, Arkansas, and had served as a guide on the White River. This was the stream where the world's record for size of both rainbow and brown trout was set. Mountain Home is a town very close to the river in the Ozark Mountains. The river had been dammed a few miles upstream, forming a very large and deep lake in Missouri. The lake was so deep at the dam site that the water issuing forth from its base was ice cold, making it an ideal habitat for trout. In addition, the state of Arkansas would stock fingerling trout every spring.

This student had his own boat and motor, and he introduced me to trout fishing. Trout normally feed on salmon eggs in their normal habitat, but there are not a lot of coastal salmon in the Ozark Mountains. Through the years, the natives in the area had found that anything yellow works wonderfully well for bait. They used canned yellow whole corn on a small hook for the rainbows and wads of cheese for the browns. Dick took me and my boys fishing a lot of times, and I can't remember a time when we didn't catch fish.

In the winter, there was no fishing the shallow rapids, as is done in the warmer weather. Dick would turn the boat sidewise to the rapid current, and we would go gliding down the crystal clear water, which was just above freezing temperature, with our corn-baited hooks trailing behind. It was dreadfully cold, but the boys never complained—though I am sure they were freezing. A rainbow trout in their grasp every so often would make them forget the discomfort.

There was another stream where we were given the pleasure of fishing. There is a tiny creek that empties into the White River named Cripple Creek. This remarkable stream is only ten- to twelve-feet wide in its widest points, and it is bone-dry in every season except spring. In the springtime, this creek is suddenly filled with rapidly-flowing water that fills it to its banks, and it is occupied by smallmouth bass in enormous numbers. The fisherman puts the john boat in upstream and floats down rapidly on the current, using the motor only to guide the boat. As he zips past the scenery, he casts lures underneath overhanging tree limbs and catches one- to two-pound, smallmouth bass. It's great fun, but I really don't think that Nancy liked it too well. Dick was yelling too many orders to everyone on her single trip.

The fishing definitely kept me from going berserk from boredom, when I suddenly got a terrific inspiration. We were seeing a number of deaf-blind babies in the clinic, and there was no facility in the immediate geographical area where we could refer them. I started looking into facilities for these children, and I found that there were only two recognized programs of excellence in the United States. One was Perkin's Institute in Boston, and the other was the School for the Deaf and Blind in Talladega, Alabama. Well, there certainly seemed to be plenty of room for another, and I began to look into what was required.

I went to a conference on the subject somewhere in Dallas, Texas. I was busily trying to decide whether to try to establish a program for Arkansas when I encountered Storm Whaley, vice president and head of the University of Arkansas Medical Center in Little Rock. We chatted for a few minutes about why I was there and he left, and I didn't see him again at the meeting. I went back home and started visiting some of the other state universities about participating in a program for deaf-blind children. Soon the question became moot, when the development of an effective vaccine against German measles was announced. This effectively canceled the need for a large deaf-blind program, as essentially all such babies are caused by the mother having rubella in the first trimester of her pregnancy.

Then I got a call one day from Storm Whaley's office, asking me to stop by for a chat. I said, "I would be happy to come, when would you like for me to drop by?"

His secretary answered me with, "How about right now?" I went down and Storm explained to me that he wanted to create a new position, assistant vice president for health affairs. This individual's purpose would be to get the medical center involved in the medical care in the state, and also help insure good patient care in the medical center. He just wanted me to think it over. He indicated to me that he had talked to several people at Alabama, and they had recommended me highly for the job. I went downstairs and talked with Ted about it, and then talked it over with Nancy. Suddenly, I again got that calm assurance feeling that this was the right thing to do. I was beginning to wonder if I wasn't fooling myself about this calm assurance thing.

Everyone seemed pleased with the appointment except one—yep, you guessed it, the head of surgery. He made a special trip to see me and to tell me that I shouldn't plan on changing a lot of things in surgery as I had done in the pediatric clinic. It would have been nice to start a new position without someone being blatantly hostile towards me. I let him rant and rave for a while, and then I told him that I had a lot to do, and I was sure that it would be a good while before I got around to surgery. With that, he huffed and puffed and stormed out of my office, grumbling and mumbling something. Surgeons depend a lot on their irascible personality in negotiations, and they really don't know what to do when you are not cowed.

At the time there was no hospital director, and I was put in his very nice office. It was a roomy corner office with large picture windows on two walls. There was a large anteroom with two secretaries at their desks. Everyone seemed to be pleased to have someone at least acting like they were in control. I put the need for a hospital administrator at the top of my list of things to do, but first I had the small financial problem of the hospital being in the red which, by state law, was illegal.

To understand this problem one must understand the state of Arkansas. The population is about equal to Alabama, except the state has only about half the space. However, Arkansas has the same number of counties, leaving it with a lot of small counties in area and no large cities other than Little Rock. Every county is absolutely filled with towns having a population of five hundred to fifteen hundred. The laws are set up so that everything of a legal nature has to be approved by the county judge. When elected, he or she is able to function as a dictator of a small county in Arkansas.

The University Hospital takes care of all the hospitalized indigent patients in the state. The process that was being followed when I looked at it showed the patients were sent to us by the local attending physician, and they would be admitted to the hospital. When they were discharged, the hospital bill was sent to the county judge's office for payment. Some would be paid and some wouldn't; it depended on the whim of the county judge. How they decided which patient's bill they were going to pay, and which they were not going to pay apparently was decided by an Ouija board or something similar. It doesn't take many such patients and, fairly soon, the hospital is developing a serious deficit.

The hooker was that, by state law, the university had to take these patients and had no right of refusal of the referral by the attending physician. There also was no recourse of appeal if a county judge says, "No." We were just supposed to find some way of paying for them. It dawned on me that the patients who were to be sent for evaluation and treated should be triaged by both the county judge and the referring physician as to whether they needed to be seen by us. If the two of them clear a patient for referral to us, then the judge would be liable for the bill. If he or she wanted to control the money, then he or she would have to make the hard decisions.

I took this plan to Storm, and he thought it would work. He called a press conference for the next day and announced the new policy. The county judges reacted in a unified way: essentially they were all irate. The newspapers ran articles about the skullduggery that was apparently going on at the university so that we were not required to accept poor, indigent patients. After having been the victim of more than a few such incidences, a person loses any absolute faith in the printed media word that he or she might otherwise have had. Storm was a very good politician, and he handled all such unfounded rumors. In a short while the hospital was solvent again, and no patient went without medical care. Miracle of miracles, the judges always found the money to pay for it.

Before I could get started finding a hospital administrator, I got a letter in the mail from the nation of Ceylon (it is now known as Sri Lanka). It was a letter from the president of the Ceylonese Academy of Pediatrics. The *Ship Hope* had been in Ceylon for the previous year, and because of the Academy's contact with American pediatrics by way of the ship, they wanted to extend an invitation to me to be the first American to give the keynote address for their national meeting. Previously, they always had invited Russian or British pediatricians. The crew from the *Ship Hope* had recommended me for the honor.

It didn't take Nancy and me long to decide we were going to accept the invitation. We went to a local travel agent who was very knowledgeable about Ceylon and eager to please. He informed us that the fare for the roundtrip would be less if we stayed at least three weeks. We could spend our extra time visiting other sites, with only the cost of meals and hotels for the extra time. That also was too good to turn down, so the agent drew up an itinerary for us. We flew to New York and took an overnight flight to Athens, Greece. We were there for two days, and spent the first morning sleeping late to help rid ourselves of jet lag. Room service brought us up Grecian coffee that was black as the ace of spades but did not taste strong. It was accompanied by hard-crusted rolls which were warm to the touch.

That afternoon we caught a cab to the Parthenon. The enormity of the place was astonishing, as was the Temple of the Vestal Virgins. Some of the huge columns had fallen, causing their separation into their component parts. Visitors could see the fluted columns were just stacks of carved marble pieces about eighteen inches in height, with a square hole cut into the center. Some type of a three-inch square rod was driven into the square holes to secure them into a column. I took detailed pictures of this construction so Pap could see how they were built.

That night, the hotel desk clerk recommended a restaurant which was located at the base of the hill housing the Parthenon. We caught a cab out there and had to walk a flight of stairs to get to the dining area. We were greeted by the maître d' whom we noticed greeted each couple in the language of the land from which he somehow discerned they hailed. He hadn't missed a one until he came to us and greeted us in French.

The view of the Acropolis from the restaurant was awe-inspiring. The entire wall facing the Parthenon was glass, allowing an unobstructed view of all the grounds and the buildings on the top and sides of the hill. It was bathed in bright light from numerous enormous floodlights. We had a delicious meal of Greek food, while at the same time enjoying this beautiful panorama.

The next morning, we had to rise before daylight and catch our flight to Colombo, Ceylon.

We landed at the Colombo airport and were greeted by our assigned hosts. They were a pediatrician and his wife, who would see to our comfort throughout our visit. They felt compelled to tell us they were Christians, which made up only ten percent of the population. The most common religion was Buddhist, and the second was Hindu. Everyone we met spoke excellent English; after all, it had been a British colony for centuries.

They carried us to our hotel, named Hotel Tappabain, and we checked into our suite, no less. The hotel was obviously an old English building, and it was filled with Victorian antiques. They still had a manually operated elevator, which was run by a short, little bronze-colored man with steel-gray hair and dressed all in white, with the white Hindu *kepi*. He would greet us when we got on the elevator by coming to attention and giving a snappy British-style salute, with the palm turned outward, followed by a "Good morning, *Sahib*." What was truly amazing about this fellow were his bare feet. I am sure that he had never worn shoes at any time in his life. His feet were about six- or seven-inches long, and about four- or five -inches wide, and his toes splayed out; so that both the little toe and his big toe pointed in opposite forty-five-degree angles. The calluses on the soles must have been at least one-half-inch thick. It is easy to see how these people could walk on broken glass or hot coals. There could not be any sensory nerve fibers anywhere close to the surface, and it would take a mighty blow and a sharp nail to get anything to pierce that callous.

Each day, we were shown around Colombo by our very gracious hosts, who tried mightily to find some Ceylonese food that we could comfortably eat. We both loved curried food, but they cooked with so much of it that neither Nancy nor I could manage the heat. The country even smelled like curry. Our hosts finally arrived at feeding us a dish they called string hoppers. It looked like white spaghetti, but it was flavored with a milder curry. It was still hot by our standards, but we could eat it without a gallon of water to keep the heat under control.

When we went out of town, we were accompanied by a young couple from the high caste of Ceylon. This was my first taste of the caste system that has ruled the society of Ceylon and India for generations. One is born into one of three social castes and remains there with no hope of moving upward in society. The boy in our traveling duo was the son of the governor of Ceylon. That is the equivalent of being the son of our president.

One evening, we were invited to a reception by the governor at his state home. It is located in downtown Colombo and built with no lawn, but it adjoined the front sidewalk. There was a covered driveway that allowed a car to get off the street and passengers to get out of a car without getting drenched during the monsoon season. There was an absolutely enormous chandelier in this parkway, filling the entire ceiling space of this covered parking area. It was constructed of metal and had at least four tiers of lamps. The lights were located at the end of long arms, and the chandelier was about twelve feet in diameter. The arms were filled with many different kinds of birds, who used the fixture as a roost.

This was not a large social event, but merely to fulfill a social obligation of welcoming us to Ceylon. The governor was a very sociable person and was dressed in the toga-like drapes of the Hindu, exhibited by Gandhi. His son, on the other hand, dressed in western garb. We sat in his study at the governor's palace and sipped squash. This wasn't something made from our yellow butternut squash, but it was something akin to drastically watered down orange juice. It was ghastly to my taste, but it did serve to prevent dawdling over a drink. Everywhere we went, we were served the same concoction. As we chatted in the study, I could not help but notice the many photographs of the governor and Mao Tse Tung scattered around the room. Later, back in my office in Little Rock, the CIA agent who came to talk with me about my trip was exceedingly curious about those photographs. During those years of the Cold War, anyone traveling out of the country who had any conversation with anyone associated with that government was visited by the CIA regularly upon returning to see if the traveler had seen or heard anything that might give any clue as to communist activity there.

The next day, our young couple drove us in a large Mercedes sedan to Kandy, a small city in the high mountains where Ceylonese tea is grown; it is the home of the Temple of the Tooth. On the way up into the mountains, we noticed that the population pretty much took up all the room available in the countryside. There were just wall-to-wall people everywhere. We saw elephants being used by the timber business to carry logs. The elephant would wrap his trunk around a good-sized log and place it on his tusks. Then he would wander on down to place the log in the desired spot while being steered by the driver astride his back, just behind his ears. He directed the animal with taps on its head with a small, thin stick. These drivers took very good care of their elephants, and they could often be seen standing in knee-deep water in a small stream, scrubbing away on the elephant's skin with a long handled brush.

Also along the way, we passed workers replanting rice plants in the rice paddies. The Ceylonese do not like American long-grained rice, but preferred a short, fat rice grain shaped like a rugby ball. This type of rice requires the seedlings to be hand-planted in dirt under about a foot of water. The soil is plowed with a plow pulled by a water buffalo who apparently doesn't mind sloshing through water while pulling that plow. One could drive past these paddies where the water buffalo would be grazing on the grass and the workers would be bent over at the waist, reaching under the water to painstakingly plant each seedling very close together. I couldn't imagine how their backs stood it.

We drove on up to Kandy and were taken to the tea plantations, where the workers were growing tea plants on mountainsides that were so steep there was no hope of mechanization. Herds of workers scoured the mountainsides and laboriously handpicked tea leaves from the mother plant, carefully placing them in a small bag strung around their neck. When the bags were full, the leaves were strewn across a wire mesh and allowed to dry on long racks in a flimsy building that was open on both ends. This would not be my favorite way to make a living.

After a light lunch we were carried to the Temple of the Tooth, where the governor's son spoke with Lamas about showing us through the temple.

The Temple of the Tooth is so named because they have one of Buddha's teeth encased in seven nested, silver caskets and kept in a crypt in the dark innards of the direct center of the building. When one enters the Temple into the area where the people come to worship, the smell of flower scents is almost overwhelming. Wild flowers, such as fragrant orchids, grow wild and abundantly throughout the entire country. These are picked by the Buddhist populace and are brought as offerings to Buddha. The monks carried us down to the tomb where the nested caskets were kept. They showed us to a small room with a doorway that was built with silver casework and a highly engraved silver doorsill that rose about a foot from the floor.

We were required to remove our shoes before entering. I stepped over the sill, but Nancy, being shorter in stature, had to step directly on the sill to get into the room. This created a furor among the monks, and they kept pointing to the sill and speaking rapidly in some tongue that definitely was not English. Apparently we had committed a major boo-boo, but after profuse apologies, everyone calmed down.

Once every year the caskets are taken outside, placed on the back of an elephant, and there is a huge parade. Apparently this is a tradition that has occurred every year for generations. I don't know how long it has been since anyone has looked into the innermost seventh casket to see if there is a tooth still there.

After the temple we were carried to the Royal Gardens, which are supposedly world renowned. They are truly lovely. The part that I enjoyed was the part of the gardens that housed the spice trees. They have every spice tree known in the world growing in the garden. It was here that I learned that allspice is a tree unto itself. Up until that time, I thought it was just a mixture of all kinds of spices.

We finished the tour with a trip out to the Governor's summer palace. This place is like something out of a movie set. In fact, it has been used as a set to film a respectable number of movies. He one that sticks in my mind was *Elephant Walk* starring Elizabeth Taylor. Her sadistic husband had built their palatial home right over the path that the elephants used every so often for some sort of migration. Naturally, the enraged elephants trampled the entire thing, including a beautiful staircase, down. A huge entrance hall is visible upon entering the front door. In the absolute center of the hall, there is a beautiful stairway, about twelve feet in width, which reaches upward to end in the center of the second floor. This has been used in innumerable movies and has been called the most beautiful stairway in the world. I was relieved to see that the elephants hadn't really done the staircase in. The stairs are constructed of dark wood, probably Ceylonese ebony, which today cannot be bought because of its rarity.

We were present just at dusk, and suddenly out of the surrounding forests came literally thousands of flying creatures winging over the clearing surrounding the castle. These were fox- eared bats that came out every evening to fly around. It is difficult to imagine the enormity of this scene, with the sky almost obliterated from sight. These flying mammals are fairly large for bats, with a wingspan of about a foot. They are protected by law and don't cause problems for the populace, since they eat only wild bananas.

The following day we were invited to the American Embassy for lunch. The embassy is a large, one-story building with a wide roof overhang topping the wide porch that surrounds the front and sides of the structure. The home is furnished with what they call Dutch furniture. It resembles our campaign furniture and is made of teak, with highly polished brass fittings. At the time we were there, the American Ballet was touring the country and they joined us at the luncheon. I was seated next to the manager of the company, and we were making small talk, as one does when there is little one has in common. He asked me in what part of America I lived. I told him that I was currently living in Arkansas, but I called Alabama home.

He said, "I have an aunt who lives in Alabama."

I replied, "Oh, really? Where does she live?"

He answered, "Fairhope." I thought, what a coincidence; I have come halfway around the world to have lunch with a fellow whose aunt lives in the same town as my parents.

My talk was anticlimactic to the visit. I gave it in a large auditorium with a great attendance. My talk was on bleeding problems in patients with gram negative septicemia. It seemed to be well received. I don't know if they have invited an American to speak again. I would hate to think that I was the first and the last.

The next morning, we made a short flight over to Bombay, India. We caught a bus in to the hotel, and it allowed us the opportunity to see Bombay arising for the morning. I found that I had misjudged Ceylon about being so crowded. Compared to Bombay, Ceylon was blessed with wide open spaces and very few inhabitants. Bombay was so crowded with the homeless that in order for everyone to have space to lie down and sleep on the street, people had to lie perpendicular to the buildings. As we looked down on the early stirring of homeless people from the vantage of our bus, we could see them walk down to the edge of a fairly wide stream, pull down their pants and urinate and defecate into the water. At the same time around a curve downstream, we could see people bathing; and further downstream around a bend were people dipping water out of the stream for drinking or cooking.

The hotel where we stayed was again an obvious holdover

from the days of the British Empire. It was a stately old red brick building with all the pomp and circumstance. We checked into a very comfortable room and then had a delicious meal in the hotel dining room while listening to a Dixieland band. We went to our room after dinner, watched an American TV show and went to sleep. We arose the next morning, went to the airport and caught a plane to Nairobi, Kenya. We didn't delve too much into the study of Indian culture.

We arrived at Nairobi in the middle of the day and caught the bus into town. This was a small bus, and there were six or seven couples on it. Each of us gave the name of our hotel, and the driver began to drop us off, one couple at a time. Most of the stops were at high-rise, modern buildings, and as we moved into the older part of town we were the only couple left. We finally stopped at this obviously old hotel made of dark-red brick. The rooms, in one-story bungalows, were scattered over a large, well groomed lawn with many shade trees. The brick bungalows were two residential units in a single building and very fashionably furnished.

Dinner was served in the hotel dining room, and they required that coat and tie be worn before getting served. Our first night, the maître d' was in a debate with a prospective diner as to whether a coat, while wearing a turtleneck shirt was sufficiently dressed to be allowed into the dining area. As I remember, the maître d' relented, but only for that single night. Unfortunately, the food wasn't comparable to the atmosphere. It was typical bland British cuisine that tasted as if it were all boiled, sans seasoning.

The next morning, we were awakened to all this jabbering going on outside our window. It was then that we learned that this was the hotel where all of the safaris were formed, outfitted with gear and safari personnel. The jabbering was from the safari workers lolling around before getting ready to depart. For a moment, I thought I was back in the emergency room in Birmingham, listening to the jabbering going on outside the entrance of the E.R. on a Friday night. The hotel was also directly across the street from the campus of the University of Kenya. The entire setting was like that of some books I had read as a youngster.

When we checked into our hotel, we were given a complimentary copy of the local newspaper. It was kind of like reading the weekly *Amory-Advertiser* of my youth, with very little national coverage, but filled with news of who was visiting whom. On the front page was a story of a train derailment just outside Nairobi. Apparently this train runs once a week, and the week prior to the derailment the train had hit an elephant and knocked him off the tracks. He got up immediately and trotted off. This week, in the same area along the tracks, as the engine puffed along an elephant came charging out of the brush, hit the engine with his head, and knocked it off the tracks. I have always heard that an elephant never forgets.

We strolled around town and then decided that we would rent a car and drive out to the game preserve outside town. We walked over to the Hertz Rental and rented a Volkswagen Beetle. The people in Kenya drive on the left side of the road, so the car's steering wheel was on the right and I had to shift gears with my left hand. I didn't really have too much difficulty driving on the left side of the road, but I do admit to getting more than a few startled looks when I made a left turn and found myself in the right lane, facing traffic.

We made it out to the game preserve without difficulty, and just as we turned into the park a huge eland stood there gazing at us. They are the largest antelopes and have spiraled, straight horns. The horns were glistening, and he was immobile while we clamored out of the car and got a picture. There were no paved roads in the park and no signs to direct traffic. The preserve is considered just a little place, but it stretches for miles. People who live on the outskirts of town have tall fences in an attempt to prevent lions from eating their pets. We really enjoyed driving around in the preserve, where the one-lane dirt roads just meander through the rolling, grassy countryside. We saw only one lion on our many trips, and that occurred when a lioness raised her immense head out of high grass located just next to the Volkswagen.

There was a small stream in a low area of the preserve which acted as a watering hole for the animals. Signs were posted everywhere, warning us to watch out for crocodiles. There were trees and underbrush going right up to the water, and it would be very easy for one of those reptiles to lie in wait for a walking morsel of food. There were also large numbers of giraffes, zebras, and different species of antelopes. All in the trees, and also walking around, were large baboons.

Baboons can be very mean animals, and they have massive jaws lined with wicked-looking teeth. Nancy was carrying a large straw purse, with the top not closed in any way, and suddenly one the brazen baboons walked up to her and grabbed her purse. This became a huge tug-of-war between Nancy and the baboon. Finally, the baboon gave a big yank and pulled the open purse to him. He held the purse open, peered down into the depths of the purse, which held our passports by the way, and after thoroughly looking, he let go, turned, and strode away in apparent disdain. Nancy recovered the purse and our passports. I thought it was funny, but Nancy sees no humor in it to this day.

On another drive through, we happened upon a lady with three children stalled along the road with a flat tire. We pulled up behind her, stopped, and I got out of the car. I asked her if I could help and put her spare tire on the car for her. She thanked me profusely, and then turned to the children and in a clipped British accent said, "Children, this nice man is going to fix our tire. Now, you watch out very carefully for lions." You've never seen a tire changed any faster in your life.

In a few days, we decided to drive north of Nairobi to Tsavo Game Park and spend a few days. It is an absolutely enormous game park with huge herds of animals. The lodging accommodations were in a stockade sort of arrangement with a large compound of low, yellow stone buildings, surrounded by an immense stone fence about twelve-feet high and about three-feet thick. There was one large gate that was closed at dusk and not opened again until dawn. Stone bungalows had very comfortable rooms that sat above the surrounding terrain on a level with the top of the fence. Along the side of the bungalow, built along the fence, were French doors opening upon a small, narrow balcony. If we strolled out on the balcony, there in all its majesty was Mount Kenya, with its snow-covered cone top.

The main building contained the administrative offices and a large covered dining area overlooking a large watering hole at the bottom of a long, gentle slope tapering downhill to the water. Lights were turned on at night, and while we were dining, we could watch all kinds of animals coming in for a cool drink of water.

Guests checking into the lodge are given a small booklet that describes the various animals seen in the preserve, and also a few warnings. The first was to never leave your car windows open if you stopped and left the car. Monkeys would tear up the inside of the car. Another rule was to never drive up to a herd of elephants with the car pointed toward the herd. If the old bull elephant became irritated with your presence, you would never have time to back out or suddenly turn around to get away if he charged the car. They cautioned to either back in or park parallel to the herd.

The first morning, we just drove around the preserve. Ostriches and giraffes were everywhere. It quickly became evident that from a distance an ostrich looks exactly like a small acacia tree, and the large acacia trees were the exact height needed for the giraffes to feed on their leaves without the need to stretch or bend over. We stopped along the way at an immense spring. This had a water flow that was at least fifteen-feet wide and spewed water out in a magnificent cascade into a large pool of crystal clear water.

There were three hippopotami frolicking around in the water, if hippopotami can frolic. They were feeding on the vegetation in the pond. We watched them swim around in the water very gracefully. It is amazing how graceful those huge animals were in the water, and how gawky they are on land. Trees surrounded the water, but there was no underbrush. I guess the swimming vegetarians kept that under control when they were stomping around on dry land. As we approached in our Volkswagen, we noticed that another car had driven up and was parked close to ours. Then we noticed that the car windows were down, and the inside of the car was totally destroyed. Wherever there are trees in Kenya there are going to be monkeys, even if they are not evident when one looks. I hope they had insurance covering monkey vandalism.

Another day we happened along a herd of elephants with calves grazing in a large field parallel to the road. We stopped and were watching them when I happened to glance in the rearview mirror and saw this enormous bull elephant charging at us. His enormous ears were standing perpendicular to his head so that all that could be seen through the rearview mirror was head and ears. I had let the car idle, so I slipped it into gear and off we sped. I looked down at the speedometer, and we were going forty miles per hour, and that elephant was keeping up. I didn't want the elephant to think I was toying with him so I increased my speed. Remember what happened to the train that toyed with an elephant?

I have thought about these experiences in Africa off and on since then. It is amazing to me to realize everything that exists on this earth is dependent on something else dying in order to sustain their life. Some say that it is the law of the jungle, where the large and powerful dominate the small and weak and use them for their food, but this is not always true. Just think of a virus which invades a person's brain and actually becomes an integral, living part of those infected cells that make up that particular organ. The virus cannot live without being incorporated into the chromosomes as either DNA or an RNA retrovirus that causes DNA to change into the same structure as the retrovirus dictates. Without this incorporation, the virus cannot sustain itself and will die.

However, now the brain is not carrying on its normal daily functions as it should. Consequently, the infested person becomes ill with a disease known as encephalitis. These altered living parts of the cells of that brain ultimately cause the brain to die, and thus the body. The virus may not die with the body, however, if it can just entice some unwary predator to eat that infected brain. It is just that in the wilds of Africa, it is so much in evidence where every "pretty" animal that we see grazing on living vegetation is being stalked by predators as a source of their food.

When we got back to Nairobi, we turned in our car. While we were at the agency, a fellow turned in his car with the front end all bashed in. He had been attacked by a rhino.

We flew out of Nairobi at night on the way to Rome. It was just in time. I had eaten about all of Kenyan food that I could take.

We arrived in Rome early in the morning and experienced a wild ride into our hotel. It seems that Italian cab drivers spend half of their driving time with their left arm out the window, the elbow bent at a ninety-degree angle, and their fingers all gathered together at the tips. While waving this arm, a stream of Italian invective (I am sure) is hurled at some driver or hapless pedestrian. This all occurs while he is driving at a very rapid rate of speed, and he is only giving the road ahead an occasional glance. We arrived at the hotel without a coronary on my part or a wreck on the driver's part. The hotel was very nice and was located at the Spanish Steps, which meant that we were in the midst of the tourist attractions. The first thing we did after checking into the hotel was to take a walk. We stopped at the first small sidewalk café that we came to and had a BLT sandwich. Nothing has ever tasted so good. Finally, I found some food that was seasoned.

We behaved like the tourists that we were. At that time, the Italian *lira* had no value to speak of on the global market. Something would be priced ten thousand *lira*, and after the initial shock of the number of zeroes present, we would realize that it was only three or four dollars. The answer to a lady's largest fantasies is buying clothing worth some astonishing number of zeroes and realizing that she can afford it.

We rode with Cook's Tours and went to see all the sights without expending any large amount of energy. As a friend of mine, Dick Higbee, said after serving in the Occupational Army there, "Rome is a very nice city. It has fountains everywhere, with water coming out of the most interesting places."

My favorite place that we visited was the Sistine Chapel. At that time, visitors walked by priceless oil paintings and other art by the most talented artists of those times, but it was the Sistine Chapel that truly captivated me. I have always been an admirer of Michelangelo and his talents and genius expressed in his paintings, architectural designs, and, above all, his sculptural genius.

I knew enough of the history of the painting of the chapel ceiling to know that he was forced to do this by Pope Julian. He didn't particularly like painting frescoes, but he really didn't like the idea of painting frescoes over that entire high, ghastly shaped ceiling. Dormer windows projected back into the ceiling, so as to essentially block any possible continuity of mural work. The impending task was to become a toil of duty for the church and a toil of love for the church. These were the real reasons that eventually broke his reluctance and allowed him to be cajoled by Pope Julian into designing and painting that ceiling. To accomplish this work required him to work on extremely high scaffolding in order to reach the ceiling. Then, because of the almost absence of sunlight in the chapel, he had to work by candlelight, lying on his back, working with wet plaster by painting the plaster while it was still wet so as to have the paint pigments to actually become a part of the plaster on the ceiling and allow the vivid colors to be bright as long as the ceiling lasted. This labor of duty and love went on for an awfully long time, but finally was finished. From what I gathered, he and Pope Julian had a very bristly relationship and Michelangelo was not too fond of the man, even if he were the pope.

In the very center of the ceiling is a depiction of Michelangelo's idea of God. He is depicted as a very large man with flowing white hair. He is reaching over and touching Adam with the tip of his forefinger and thus giving him life. I have thought about this concept of life being given by the touch of God. In my professional life as a pediatric hematologist-oncologist, I have been present many times when children have died. Children, as a rule, don't seem to dwell on dying one way or the other. So often at the time of death, they would be looking at me without fear or agitation, and I could see the light in their eyes simply turn off. Nothing has changed physically with the child, but suddenly I could see that life as we know it is simply gone. At that time, nothing that man can do changes anything. All the hysterics of resuscitation as depicted on TV offers no benefit at all. It is much better to accept death as it comes and not subject children's bodies to man's invasive techniques. In my fifty-four years of practicing pediatrics, I have never seen one of these children resuscitated. I have often wondered if that is the time that the soul actually leaves the body.

We flew on to London, and there we also did all the tourist things. We stayed at a small hotel just around the corner from Piccadilly Square. We were in walking distance of the entire major and some minor theaters in London. We went to a play each night, and I thoroughly enjoyed every minute of it. I have always enjoyed the theater over movies or television. However, all good things must come to an end, and the day came when we motored out to Heathrow Airport and flew back to Little Rock.

After being gone for around three weeks, there was plenty of work that had been carefully saved for me. I should have remembered another piece of advice that Dr. Platou gave me. He said, "If you are going to be gone for a while, always stay long enough so problems have to be solved by someone and they can't save them until you return." The hospital administration had to be formed, so I wrote several places advertising the position. We got several applications but none that I particularly liked, so I contacted a friend of mine at Alabama. Jim Crank was second in command at University of Alabama Hospital all the time through the growing era to the time we started talking about this position. He was still young enough to have the energy for the job, and after talking for a while, he decided to come join us.

He arrived that fall and completely took the hospital off my hands. In the meantime, I found other things to keep me busy. I found out that in the smaller towns of the state, general practice physicians were having a difficult time getting their EKGs read. They were not really qualified to read them themselves, and there was always a long delay getting a qualified reading. I thought that since we were the state's hospital, there should be some way that we could offer this service to the physicians needing the help. I hit upon the idea that the EKGs could be sent by phone wires to us, and our cardiologists could read them and call a reading back immediately. I had several conferences with our cardiologists, who were very anxious to set it up.

There the enthusiasm ended. I got replies, such as the transmission of EKGs was too unreliable to be of use. This was during the moon landings, and I seized on this. I declared, "Do you mean to tell me that we are able to do an EKG of a man on the moon, and we can't transmit an EKG from West Memphis, Arkansas?" I never got that one past the state medical society.

I had other problems that I had to deal with that had nothing to do with medicine. We had an unannounced visit from a representative of the Equal Opportunity Employment Service. He was a snotty little black man who immediately rubbed me the wrong way. He pompously said, "I am here to be sure that the minorities are being hired here without discrimination."

I answered him by saying, "We hire faculty according to their abilities, not whether they are minorities or not."

He answered, "That is understood, but we need to see if you are hiring minorities."

I said, "Well, we have a full-blooded Japanese on the faculty."

He cleared his throat and said, "That is not what I am here for."

I wouldn't let it go; after all, he was acting like a first-rate jackass. So I continued, "But they are the only Japanese family in the entire area; you can't get any more minority than that." He brushed me off with some mumbled comment. I then said, "What you really want to know is how many blacks we have on the faculty." He sighed and nodded his head. Well, we had several, including Jocelyn Elders, who would later be named surgeon general of the United States by Bill Clinton. We didn't hear from them again.

We clearly had a parking problem at the medical center. The hospital and medical school sat on top of a small hill. Both buildings, plus the state psychiatric hospital, occupied the entire top of that hill. The basic science building and the hospital were joined by a crosswalk that started on the second floor. If a patient drove to the top of the hill he or she could drive under the catwalk, but there were only eight or ten parking spaces up there. For some reason, there were no parking accommodations for visitors, no matter who you were. It certainly didn't build public good will. Families of hospital patients, visitors to the outpatient clinic, and other visitors had to park on a small parking lot at the foot of the hill.

One weekend while visiting my folks, Mr. Smith, who had a bay house two houses down from Pap's, was telling me that there was a city-style bus for sale in Mobile. When I heard this, I had a brainstorm. Sitting next to the Medical Center in Little Rock is War Memorial Stadium, where the Arkansas Razorbacks played some of their football games. It had a huge parking area, and since it was a state-owned facility, we were eligible to use it for our parking needs. If we could buy this city bus, we could run a constant shuttle from the stadium to the hospital. Everyone thought it was a wonderful solution, but when I called back to Mobile it had been sold.

No one would talk to me about buying a new bus, so the idea fizzled. We continued to have problems, however, as typified by an incident with the governor, Mr. Winston Rockefeller. He visited us one day, and since there were no parking places on top of the hill, his chauffeur pulled up beside the sidewalk and parked. The governor came in, and after a short meeting he walked out and his car was gone. We asked the guard where the governor's car was and he replied, "I made the guy move it; there is no parking up here." I told him to go get the car, and in a short time the car drove up the hill, the governor got in, and it drove off.

We asked the guard why he made the governor's chauffeur move his car. He answered indignantly, "Dr. Bentley, for the money you pay me, you ain't gonna get no Paris diplomat." He made a good point. We never did get that parking problem solved while I was there.

I then got another bright idea; at least, I thought it was good. This time in history was during the Vietnam War, with daily news broadcasts on TV showing wounded soldiers being transported by helicopters to a hospital unit. Why not set up this type of program in Arkansas for accident victims needing care? These and other critical care patients, etc., could be flown into our emergency unit for rapid and skilled care. I was sure that we could get a federal grant to expand and modernize our emergency unit. The first problem was where to get helicopters. We were fortunate that a medical helicopter National Guard unit was housed in Little Rock.

I went to talk with the commanding officer of the helicopter unit, and he was all excited about participating in this program because it would allow him to keep his helicopters and pilots well trained and functioning. He was also very realistic. He told me, "I wish you good luck, but you are fighting an uphill battle. Nothing is harder to do in Arkansas than to introduce a new idea and get people to accept it. The state has an inferiority complex; they don't believe they can get anything new accomplished." Truer words were never spoken. Every time I talked to people about it, I was ridiculed. Of course, nowadays every hospital has a helipad for patients brought in by helicopters.

In those days, the University of Arkansas football team played several games at War Memorial Stadium. It apparently is a tradition that each game program for these football games include a full-page tribute to a faculty member. I don't know how they pick the member to be so honored, but I was chosen to be that person for some big game. I knew nothing about it and didn't know that I was being put in the program. The following Monday, I got a phone call from my nemesis in the surgery department. He was livid that I had been written up and was certain that I had orchestrated the whole thing. He ranted, "It makes you sound like the Second Coming." I thought that was funny, but I didn't laugh in his face. I was afraid he would burst a blood vessel. I never saw a copy of that page, but it must have been a lulu.

When I first started this job, the University Hospital had nothing to do with the other hospitals in town, Baptist and St. Vincent's hospitals. The hospital administrator at St. Vincent's Hospital was a very nice and cooperative fellow. He and I talked a lot, and we started talking about sharing programs, and thus, costs. More bangs for your buck was the whole idea. We had essentially no private patients at University except for a very few referrals. It was Alabama all over again; we needed the private patients to enlarge the scope of our teaching program.

When I talked to Baptist, it wasn't so cordial or warm. I think that Baptist Hospitals, as a rule, are hesitant to form unions for patient care. It reminds me of the joke about this fellow going to heaven. He is met by Gabriel, who acts as his personal guide to show him around. They come to this enormous room where everyone is playing bingo. Gabriel says, "Those are the Catholics." They stroll on a little further, and they come to this room having a huge "dinner on the ground." Gabriel announces, "Those are the Methodists." Continuing on, they arrive at another room filled with people enjoying a cocktail party. Gabriel speaks up again to say, "Those are the Episcopalians."

Suddenly the fellow notices a closed pair of absolutely monumental doors. He says, "What's in there?"

Gabriel puts his forefinger to his lips and says, "Shhh. That's the Baptists; they think they are the only ones up here."

Over time, we were beginning to make some headway into possibly having coordinated programs so the costly equipment could be shared. I even got to the point of looking into the feasibility of constructing a monorail connecting the three hospitals. This would solve any future parking problems, and we would be on a par with Disney World. That's about as far as I got with that one.

I had one final fling at trying to put the University of Arkansas Medical Center first in something. Back in those days, hospital computers were in their infancy. Any computer-driven programs required huge computers that would fill a large room and produce enough heat so as to require a separate air-conditioning system. There were two big companies then, IBM and CDC from California. CDC doesn't exist anymore under that name, but I don't know who bought them out. The units that we had for the lab and admitting were CDC-made equipment. One day I was chatting with the head of our computer department and a CDC representative.

The CDC representative mentioned that they were beginning to develop a program to completely computerize a hospital. Everything that was usually written on paper would be on the computer. They envisioned that it would all but eliminate clerical errors, speed up admissions and discharges, and solve the problem of physicians' undecipherable hand writing. I jumped on that one. I said, "Where are you planning on setting this up?" He said that was not decided, but wherever it was, it would cost the hospital nothing to have it installed and maintained. I knew that we could afford that. I quickly asked, "How does one apply?"

He replied, "If you are interested, why don't you visit us and we can discuss it?" I quickly accepted the invitation and found myself and three other people flying to San Diego. We rented a car and drove south to the company's headquarters. The next morning, we met with the company hierarchy until lunch. They took us to a beautifully situated restaurant, built high on a cliff above a small inlet of the Pacific Ocean. The day was cloudless and the water in the inlet was a fantastic blue, where black and white Orcas rolled on the surface. The view was better than the food, which was fabulous.

We continued meeting during the afternoon, and when we

finished, we had a solid offer from CDC to install its new hospital system in the University of Arkansas Medical Center, free of charge. CDC's only requirement was that after all the bugs had been worked out and it was functioning well, the center wanted to be able to bring in representatives from other hospitals to see how it worked. In other words, all we were required to do to obtain these thousands of dollars' worth of computer equipment and expertise was to let other people observe the working model in our hospital. I was walking on cloud nine when we left California.

The whole idea was met with total disdain by the university. All sorts of reasons surfaced, but they just weren't ready to try something with the possibility of alienating the established way of doing things. I was feeling mighty low, and it was during this time that I walked into my office and found Dr. John Simpson sitting there. He was a living symbol that you shouldn't let the inability of some people to see bigger possibilities get you down.

About this time Dr. Ted Panos, my friend and colleague, had a fatal coronary occlusion. There was a lot of speculation of my replacing him, both pro and con. I had no interest in that at all. Then in a few days, Storm Whaley called me in to say that he was accepting some kind of position in Washington, D.C. Again the speculation began again over my replacing him. I found that I had no desire to take on that job either. I felt like I had done my job that brought me here, and perhaps it was time for me to return to my original dream. Again I submitted another resignation after I secured my future in Mobile with a phone call. I said my good-byes to my friends, put my house up for sale, and moved on to southern Alabama.

Since leaving there, I have thought many times about my meeting Storm at that seminar on deaf-blind children in Dallas. Neither of us was particularly interested in the subject; in fact, I never found out what he was doing there. I was simply there to find something useful to do with my time in Arkansas; I had already taken care of the problem in the outpatient clinic.

Chapter 12

The University of South Alabama — Utter Frustration

When I decided to leave Arkansas, I thought long and hard about my future. I was getting a little long in the tooth to be thinking about starting from scratch with a solo private practice. There were still no pediatricians in Fairhope, and it would frankly take too long to establish a going practice. I didn't think that I still had enough of the vital energy it would take for that chore. So I thought that I would probably do better to join a good established group that adhered to the same principles as mine for the practice of medicine.

That is when I talked with Dr. Jim Coker, who was leaving Mobile to be the medical director of the state's Crippled Children's Service. He had practiced in Mobile since finishing his residency at Alabama, so he was very familiar with the different practices. He told me that I should contact Children's Medical Group. This was a new group formed from various private practices in the Mobile area, and it was the group that he was connected with before his present appointment with the state. He and his old partner, Hollis Wiseman, had gone in with others to originally form the group. He was leaving to take this new position because it was something that he had always wanted to do. Hollis was moving over to Mobile General Hospital to be in charge of the pediatric residency program. Bill McDaniel was leaving to do a pediatric radiology residency in Colorado. It seemed apparent that this was a very good group of doctors, and they practiced pediatrics with the highest ideals of medicine.

I had talked with John Shriner before about several things, so I gave him a ring. He was very enthusiastic about my coming down, so Nancy and I drove down. This was a group of pediatricians who had many years of pediatric experience between them. John Shriner and Bobby Harris had been partners before the merger. They were both slightly older than I. Peter Bertucci had a solo practice and was about my age. Jim Roberts had just finished his residency at Mobile General and had gone to Alabama when I had been there. He liked to tell the story about coming into my office for his oral exam in pediatrics. He claimed that I said, "Have a seat. Now tell me all you know about DiGuglialmo's syndrome." He acknowledged that I immediately said that I didn't really expect him to know that. He said that the only problem with that was he couldn't remember his name after that initial shock.

This group had very high ideals for its practice. It never closed. Even on holidays, someone was in the office during regular office hours and was on call all that night to care for the group's patients. Each physician had his own patients, and they would be seen by that person on the day they called if they had an opening. If there was no opening, the patient was seen by one of the partners if the parent was comfortable with the person. Most parents had their doctor, and they had their second-choice physician to see. After hours, the late man saw all patients by appointment that wanted to be seen.

There was no closing time for the office. The doctor went home when everyone was seen. All calls that came in during the day with parents' questions or discussions about their child were given to their physician's nurse. All of the office nurses were registered nurses, and most had many years of experience doing this. The nurses stayed along with the late physician and office help during week days. On weekends, two physicians made hospital rounds at all three hospitals for all the other physicians, seeing both the hospitalized patients and newborns. On Saturday, both physicians worked the mornings and into the afternoon if the patient load required it. The fellow who was on duty for Sunday was on second call for back up on Saturday afternoon and night. They both made rounds again on Sunday morning, but only one physician went on to the office. Sundays were usually lighter in patient load, but the Saturday man was on call as back up if patient load required it.

During the weekdays each physician saw his own hospitalized

patients and newborns at all three hospitals, unless he was off duty that day. In that case, his patients would be seen by whichever partner had patients or newborns in that same hospital. The physician on second call made afternoon rounds on any hospitalized patients that needed to be checked on. The person on duty the night prior would call each physician working that day, distribute patients to be seen, and discuss new admissions with whomever had new patients admitted. It all sounded good to me.

We agreed on a guaranteed salary until the time that I had built my practice and didn't require subsidy. We shook hands and that was it. We returned to Little Rock and made plans for moving. The business manager had found us a house to rent in the Springhill area, just a couple of blocks away from the Mobile Country Club. The only problem that we had was our big, old cat, who had adopted us when we moved into our current house. All the moving activities had scared him, and old Clarence had gone to hide. We finally found him in a storm drain opening in the street curbing, sitting on a ledge. Nancy lay on the street and coaxed him to let her pick him up. He moved with us several times after that but never seemed to be bothered by the entire moving hubbub again.

The home that we had rented was a very nice house. The lady who lived there was away at school, getting accredited for teaching deaf children. The house was fairly new and spacious. The school that the boys attended was located so they could easily walk to my office after school if need be. That gave us a year to look for a place to live. Jane Crosby was the real estate agent who suffered through the experience of trying to find us a house we both liked. We found that, although Mobile was filled with historic homes, all the houses that were for sale looked as if they had been taken straight out of *Better Homes and Gardens* magazine. It got to the point that as soon as we opened the front door, we knew exactly what the floor plan was. After many fruitless sorties searching for the right house, Jane announced that she just wasn't going to be able to find a house to suit us. She said, "I am going to introduce you to Tommy McCowan. He designs and builds houses, and I think the two of you would hit it off." And that is how our lives became entwined with Tommy.

Tommy was a native Mobilian, from one of the old Mobile families, and grew up on Government Street. He was one of the most unorthodox people I have ever known, which made him someone I really enjoyed being around. He had bright blue eyes that really did sparkle, had an almost constant grin on his face, and wore the most outlandish colors in his wardrobe of anyone I have ever been around. He had no formal architectural training, but he had an absolute marvelous talent for house design. He would envision what he wanted, and then he would get a draftsman to put the vision on paper and obtain the engineer's scrutiny to insure that it was going to be stable. He had a steady crew of finish carpenters, brick masons, etc., who built the house from scratch.

During the Depression, the government hired out-of-work architects to draw detailed plans of a great many of the old homes in Mobile for preservation purposes. A lot of those homes were torn down during the urban renewal craze of the 1950s, but those plans still exist at the Mobile Public Library. Tommy sat down with us and determined what we wanted our house to look like, and the number and size of rooms that we wanted in the house. He came back with a plan based on the house that at one time sat next to the Mardi Gras Museum on Government Street. We liked it and contracted with Tommy to build it. I obtained a construction loan, and Tommy built the house at cost plus ten percent.

That way, I got to take off enormous deductions from my income tax for sales tax paid on supplies bought for the house. The construction time exceeded the year we had in our rented house, so we moved into an apartment until we could move into our new home. It was a pleasure working with Tommy on that house. He would call me and say, "Shug (his wife) wants a new washing machine and dryer; could you leave me a check for X amount of dollars so I can keep her happy?" During the years that we lived there, I would build a lot of furniture to make it livable. It was a very comfortable home to be in.

During these years, John got immersed in Little League baseball. Our cousin, Jerry Peake, was a manager of one of the teams, and John played on his team. We never missed a game. John started out playing first base, but down the line wanted to become a pitcher. I spent a lot of late afternoons after work squatting down and having John hit the mitt. I really enjoyed all that. Paul would go with us to the park when we would be working on John's hitting or fielding, but he never showed any interest in joining a team.

I worked hard at my practice, and in a short time had built a comfortable patient following. Initially, the practice was general pediatrics, but soon not only did the referrals for hematology-oncology patients increase, but also those for patients with unusual diseases as well. Eventually, in later years, my practice became almost wholly a referral practice with all sorts of interesting patients to diagnose and to treat.

Somewhere along in here, I was asked to be a part of the visiting faculty for the California Pediatric Society yearly state meetings. They needed a hematologist to give a couple of sessions and be on some panels. Some of my friends in Minnesota had recommended me. The meetings were held in Palm Springs at one of the resorts. My talks went well, and after the first one a guy came up to speak with me. It was the fellow who replaced me at Barksdale AFB. The world remained a small place for me. This was my last talk to a large group in my career. The talks were taped by a continuing education company, and they used my talk on platelets for one of their education tapes to which the Mobile Infirmary subscribed. It came out shortly after we got back to Mobile, and that caused a little buzz amongst the medical staff. However, there were no parades or anything.

Several years before all of this was occurring, Gordon Persons, the then-governor of Alabama, and the state legislature voted for the establishment of a second medical school in the state; primarily, I think, to spite the University of Alabama. There was no stipulation as to where this school was going to be placed, and after the decision to build it became a fact, the state had to decide where to put it. This became a problem because none of the old state schools wanted it for several reasons. Chief among these was that this new school would always be the stepchild of the University of Alabama.

There is an old joke that explains it. This university President dies, and since he had not been an exemplary man, he was standing at the gates of Hell while the decision was being made as to what to do with him.

Finally Lucifer says, "We are going to make a college president out of you."

To which the subject said, "But, I already am a college president."

To this Lucifer replied, "Ah, but this one has a medical school."

After trying many different schools, the fledgling South Alabama University was given the school in an act of desperation as much as anything else. Part of this decision was because the Medical College of Alabama was originally located in Mobile before it was moved to Tuscaloosa. Anyway, that sounded good. Apparently there was some real coercion on the part of Governor Persons to get this placement agreed to and accepted.

During the time that I was building my practice, the medical school was being put together. They finally got around to appointing Dr. Bob Bucher as the first dean of the school of medicine after I was settled in at Children's Medical Group. He was brought in with the mandate to build a medical school that was closely aligned with the practicing physicians of Mobile County. It was supposed to allow students to be taught the practicalities as well as the esoterics of medicine. I thought that was a commendable effort because so many schools don't have really good clinicians on their faculties. By far, most medical school clinical faculties have never practiced a day of private practice, yet they are quick to tell everyone how it should be done. Truly, ignorance is bliss. This is the cause of the "town and gown" coldness that one sees in most medical schools. For some reason, there invariably animosity occurs between the faculty (the gowns) of a medical school and the town (the local physicians). The faculty tends to demean the medical prowess of the town, and the town physicians think the faculty knows nothing about day-to-day medical care. If they are working together, perhaps understanding of each others' medical worlds will obviate much of the hostility.

I had stayed out of all of this because I really had no interest in returning to academic medicine. I read in the local newspaper about some of the happenings, but I really was not interested in what was going on. One afternoon, as I was busily seeing patients, the girls in the reception area told me I had a call from Dr. Bucher. He introduced himself, and said that he was calling me to see if there was any interest on my part about being a part of the new medical school. He buttered me up some by telling me how respected I was in the medical and academic communities. I didn't let that go to my head, since I had done exactly the same thing too many times before.

He continued, "We are planning to set this up a little differently than the usual hierarchy arrangements of the older medical schools. I am going to set up divisions in the school consisting of several regular departments, and these division heads will be my inner council. The one that I hoped we might interest you in is what we are going to call the division of growth and development. It will include OB-GYN, medical genetics, and pediatrics. In addition to your divisional duties, you would be professor and chairman of the department of pediatrics. However, you would select and recruit the chairman of the other two departments. I would like for you to think it over, and if you have any interest, I would like an opportunity to talk with you. If you are not interested, then we need to start looking for someone else for the position." I told him that I would think it over and let him know.

I must confess to more than a little annoyance at this call. This would be getting involved in something in which I had absolutely no interest whatsoever. Here, again, was something trying to pull me away from what I wanted to do. My first inclination after ending the call was to call him back immediately and tell him I appreciated the courtesy and honor of being asked, but I was happy doing what I was doing. Then I remembered one of my mama's sayings, "Act in haste, repent at leisure." So I began to look at it as a possibility. I talked it over with my partners, and I expressed my preference for just not getting involved. They in response cautioned no rash decisions, that probably the future practice of pediatrics in Mobile would be affected greatly by this appointment.

While I was wrestling with all of this, I got another call from Bob Bucher. He just wanted to know if I had given any consideration to the position. Again, that calm hit me as before, and I told him that I would like to talk about it. We met in his office in the new school of medicine basic science building on the main campus. I laid out my plan for the pediatric department as I envisioned it, with extensive involvement of the practicing physicians. Our students, while on their pediatrics rotation, would spend a specified amount of time in the offices of our clinical faculty learning practical pediatrics, such as ear infections, rashes, etc. These instructors would submit questions to be used in their final exam. There would be a strong research component to the full-time faculty which would include the recruitment of some proven scientists. I felt that this would merge the various components of a pediatric department into the best overall whole that we could muster for a brand-new school. Bob liked every bit of it, and as I had done so many times previously with other bosses to be, we shook hands.

I worked out my arrangement with Children's Medical Group that I would continue my working there, but in a smaller capacity. All of my hematology-oncology patients were to be seen there, and my office nurse would be paid out of my pediatric department account. I would take my regular night-call rotation, but would take no more newborn patients. My money earned in the practice would pay all the overhead for my practicing there, and the remainder would be placed in a pediatric account at the university that was under strict control of university regulations.

Now I had the problem of what to do about people who were previously working for Mobile General and who had no position in the medical school. There always seemed to be some individuals left over from previous arrangements who were miffed that they didn't get my job. This held true with this position. This individual was a well-trained pediatric generalist who was born and raised in Mobile; at one time, he had an active private pediatric practice and recently had been director of the Pediatric Residency program at Mobile General Hospital. In his pediatric practice, he had cared for the University President's children, and he and the President of the University had become friends. Later, he would utilize this friendship to its utmost in an effort to undermine pediatric policies and advance his own agenda. All of this, in his mind, should have made him the logical choice to be the new Chairman of Pediatrics. He didn't hesitate to tell me that very fact. As the immortal Yogi Berra once said, "It's déjà vu all over again."

I pretty much just ignored that outburst. Another of my mother's adages was, "Least said, the least mended." I responded by saying, "You look at all the positions open in a pediatric department, including the nurseries, and I will recommend you for a professor position in charge of whatever you want to do." He eventually chose the newborn nurseries since, as you may remember, they had been recently built and paid for by the public health grant we used to build the program in Birmingham. I finally received some fruit from my past toils.

The department of genetics was my next task. I was in familiar territory; pediatricians who were well trained in pediatric medical genetics were a rare breed. I called the pediatric geneticist at John Hopkins. I had known him for several years, and we had him down to Alabama as a visiting faculty member for one our postgraduate education programs. I asked him to recommend someone for this post. I told him that we needed a real geneticist and not someone who just grew chromosomes and called himself a geneticist. Growing chromosomes and matching up the pairs was the latest fad in medicine at that time.

He recommended a fellow up at Harvard named Wladimir Wertelecki. I found that Wladimir was a very unusual fellow. He was born in the Ukraine and lived there until a small boy. This was during the reign of Stalin, who I surmise was not a family favorite. His father died when Wladimir was around six, as I understand. What part the controlling regime had to do with it, I don't know. At any rate, his remaining family had to flee the country and wound up in Spain. Wladimir went to school there, and in self-defense had to learn Spanish. Later, they moved to Portugal, then France, and eventually moved to South America.

He got his MD degree in Argentina, and moved on to America at Washington University in St. Louis. He says that at that time he had a very thick, guttural Russian accent. He went to the speech and hearing department and asked them to help him get rid of his accent. At first they refused to consider it, but he argued that they helped cleft palate patients and those with other things, like lisps, speak well. He won the argument, and they began to work on his accent. He received a position at NIH and had to leave before they completely rid him of an accent, but he barely had one when I met him. He was fluent in six languages by the time I tracked him down up at Harvard.

We corresponded several times, and he and his wife came down for a visit. We sold them on the idea of joining us. By that time we had moved into a metal building behind the Mobile General. However, I guess by that time the name had been changed to University Hospital. Our spacious quarters for our division provided room for the needed laboratory facilities and offices for the new department of medical genetics.

Along with this, I had to find a chairman for the OB-GYN department. I appointed a search committee consisting of local obstetricians and faculty members and told them to start looking. I reminded them that it had to be someone who would be comfortable with the local physicians and who would not create a "town and gown" situation. They eventually recommended a fellow out in California, Hi Mendenhall, who had both an active practice in obstetrics and an academic background. We invited him to visit, and while he was here we had dinner at Constantine's, a very fine old Mobile restaurant.

We were having a pleasant meal when someone said something about Dr. Bentley. Our waitress, who appeared to be an older lady, stared at me and said in a voice that could be heard over the entire restaurant, "Are you Dr. Herschel Bentley?"

In a much quieter tone, I answered, "Yes, I am."

Then in the same high volume tone she screamed, "Why, you saved my granddaughter's life!" I asked her who her granddaughter was, and she told me in a much quieter voice. It is true that I had saved her granddaughter's life by diagnosing a very rare type of anemia and successfully treating it when she was an infant. Now everyone in the restaurant knew it. It was an embarrassing moment for me, as I don't like to attract attention to myself. The dinner progressed without further accolades and the waitress refused a tip. While we were eating, Hi mentioned that his practice partner was a graduate of the University of Alabama's School of Medicine. After pinning it down, I discovered that his partner was a classmate of mine named Bill Hammack. It continued to be a small world.

Hi went on to build a very fine department with an excellent clinical faculty and an active residency program. However, in a short time after moving here with his family, his wife contracted a fatal illness and died. He became deeply depressed, and despite all the medical and social help that could be offered, he died. I truly think he lost his will to live without his wife.

It was time now to build another department of pediatrics. I made a conscious decision to recruit older, more established, faculty members rather than the approach I used at Alabama of risking young, upcoming faculty whom we expected to bloom into exceptional faculty members. The first person that I got in touch with was Dr. Ray Peterson, who had been chief pediatric resident when I was in Minnesota. He had been a fellow with Bob Good and was also a Guggenheim Fellow at Upsala University in Sweden. He felt right at home there, as his grandparents were immigrants from Sweden to the United States. He had distinguished himself with his immunologic work and his research in leukemia. He became my right-hand man. He moved his wife and three kids down when the boys were of the age to be in junior high and high school. That is not a good time to be uprooted, as I can attest. I don't think that any of the family approved the move except Ray.

I also added an endocrinologist from Arkansas, a gastroenterologist from California, and started looking for an infectious disease person. Later, I would try to recruit Jocelyn Elders to join us. She was an excellent endocrinologist, and at that time was in charge of all of the pituitary growth hormone in the United States. In fact, I had a young boy referred to me from Atmore, Alabama, with an extremely small stature. We determined that he did not make growth hormone and could be labeled a hypopituitary dwarf. Growth hormone was a very scarce commodity then, as it was derived solely from pituitary glands obtained at autopsy. I called Jocelyn, who had me fill out all sorts of forms, and after assurances that the boy would be followed in the recommended manner I got the growth hormone. He was followed by the endocrinologist in the department and grew five inches the first year. He is now a normal-sized individual, as far as I know, and has very grateful parents.

We invited Jocelyn to visit, but her joining us was complicated by the fact that her husband was a high school basketball coach and would need a job. Try as I might, I couldn't pull that one off. Jocelyn stayed at Arkansas, and somehow got involved with the Clintons when Bill was governor. When he became president, he appointed Jocelyn as Surgeon General. That appointment didn't work out well, and she subsequently returned to Arkansas. I haven't seen her since.

We had fifteen students in the first class to reach the third year. That allowed us to evaluate the program and to put medical students for a short rotation in the private pediatricians' office. It went extremely well, and we continued that practice until a new Dean stopped it. That's another story that we'll cover later. Every morning, the students assigned to the wards, the ward house staff, and I met to discuss new admissions from the day before. The admitting resident presented the patient, and this was followed by a detailed discussion of the presenting symptoms and the physical diagnosis. This was not a grilling of the resident, but we talked about what the symptoms suggested was wrong, what the resident would expect to see on physical exam, and the proof or disproof of the clinical impression by what the laboratory findings were.

Just like Dr. Harrison before me, I expected any laboratory data to be obtained with the aim of ruling diseases in or out. In short, I wanted them to learn to have a good differential diagnosis made and the list shortened by physical exam and further defined by lab work. These were popular sessions with both the students and the house staff. Once a week, the ward residents, the head of the pediatric nursing service and I met to discuss any complaints from students, house staff or visiting or permanent faculty as to problems encountered on the ward the previous week. As Dr. Platou taught me, no complaint was addressed unless it was presented in writing.

Ray and I began to merge our work in leukemia in children.

We wanted to be able to prove the etiology of acute lymphocytic leukemia, which was the most common type of leukemia seen in children. Ray had already been actively working with chicken leukemia. First, here are a few basic facts about what we knew from previous work by Ray, Bob Good and others.

Bob showed that there were two major types of lymphocytes in the body. One type is B cells, so named because of work done at Mississippi State University by Dr. Bruce Glick, showing that the lymphocytes that actively make antibodies in the chicken come from a small sac of lymphocytes which are located off the lower end of a chicken's intestinal tract. He named them B cells for bursa, and when it was found that B cells existed in humans and any other animals that were tested the same nomenclature was kept. If these types of lymphocytes become malignant, then it is a slow-growing type mainly seen in adults, and it is called chronic lymphatic leukemia. Usually something else kills the patient before this type of leukemia does, as it has a life expectancy of fifteen to twenty years when it is untreated.

The other type of lymphocyte seen is solely made by the thymus gland, which dictates the production of antibody-producing lymphocytes. Bob Good was the investigator who proved their role in the immune system. These cells, named T cells because of their origin in the thymus gland, cause B cells to be made that produce a specific antibody. If a patient has an illness that requires antibodies is immunized against a certain organism such as mumps or measles, the T cells are manufactured so as to immediately recognize the invading bacterium, virus, etc. Theoretically, if the patient again comes in contact with that organism, one or more T cells that are programmed to recognize that particular antigen are activated, and by cloning make many more identical T cells. They in turn stimulate the cloning of B cells in the regional lymph nodes to make antibodies to that organism. Thus a person is apt to experience enlarged regional lymph nodes such as in the neck with strep throat. It is all supposed to work that way. If T cells become malignant, this is called acute lymphocytic (or lymphoblastic) leukemia.

All species of animals with active immune systems may develop acute lymphocytic leukemia. The cause of leukemia in almost all such animals, except the human, has been shown to be viral infections. There are only two animals that have horizontal transmission of leukemia; that is, they are contagious. These are chickens and cats. Chickens have both T cell and B cell leukemia. Epidemics of leukemia were a plague for people in the poultry business, as one or the other type would move in and decimate a poultry farmer's flocks. These are prevented from occurring nowadays. Cats transmit leukemia virus readily, and it has been demonstrated that if cats live in a cattery, thirty percent will develop leukemia.

All other animals have been shown to have vertical transmission of a virus. That is, the virus is transmitted to offspring as an inherited strip of a chromosome. When an embryo is developed after fertilization of the egg by sperm, the embryo contains the leukemia virus if it existed as part of the mother's or father's DNA. That leukemia virus becomes a live and integral part of the embryo's immune system. If something stimulates the replication of a specific T cell to increase the production of viral contained T cells, they apparently will grow in a rampant fashion with no obvious control system, and a malignant bone marrow results. The question then becomes, Why do these T cells continue to grow in a totally uncontrolled manner after receiving a seemingly normal call for the production of these cells? They were solely stimulated to subdue some occurrence that called for the production of a large number of T cells.

In the 1930s, the Nobel Prize was awarded to an investigator who took ovaries from female rats and made a small incision into the same rat's spleen, where he tucked the ovary and sutured the spleen closed. The ovary would live in such an environment because of the large blood pool always present in a spleen. Normally, under stimulus from the pituitary gland, if the blood level for the estrogen hormone is low, the ovary is stimulated to make estrogen. The pituitary gland cuts off its stimulation when the estrogen level reaches normal values. It works like the thermostat in your house: if it gets cold, the thermostat turns the heat on; and when the house warms up, the thermostat turns the heat off.

However, in this circumstance, the estrogen level falls because the ovary, though living in the body, cannot put estrogen into the blood stream since it has neither venous nor arterial direct connections. Thus there is a situation where an organ is constantly being stimulated to produce estrogen; but, try as it might, the ovary cannot effectively cause any estrogen to reach the circulation. After a period of time the ovary was removed, and lo and behold, the ovary had become malignant. This is known as a hormonal malignancy or a cancer caused by the over stimulation of a hormone.

In earlier times, a researcher named Dr. Ludwig Gross believed that essentially all malignancies were caused by the vertical transmission of cancer-causing viruses. This was not a popular thought in those days, and Dr. Gross told me that when he would enter a room, individuals would get up and leave. He was trying to work with a virus that caused leukemia in a certain strain of rats, but he was having no success causing leukemia by injecting his virus into young rats. They seemed to thrive on it. One day, he went to a lecture being given at the university on the immune system in the rat. The lecturer made a statement that rats developed an active immune system in just a few days after birth and were able to reject any viral infections, unless they were given in just a short time after birth. Ludwig said he leapt up out his seat and literally ran to his lab because he had a rat that delivered a litter of young that very morning. He injected all of the litter with his virus, and in six weeks they all had leukemia. He had proven his point. He was no longer a simple-minded outcast, but a brilliant investigator who had made an extremely important discovery.

Ray got Dr. Gross to send us some of his Gross virus in the form of organs from rats with leukemia. We extracted the virus according to Dr. Gross's instructions, injected them into baby, newborn rats' bellies, and we had rat leukemia galore.

The thymus makes T cells as its function in life. It is stimulated to make T cells by a stimulus from a hormone named thymosin. We reasoned if leukemia were a hormonal malignancy, then it had to be because the pituitary gland was making excess thymosin, thus stimulating the manufacture of T cells. Since the thymus couldn't respond normally and stop the stimulation of massive hordes of T cells, just like the ovary tucked away in that rat's spleen, the thymus gland started making T cells uncontrollably. This is leukemia—acute lymphoblastic leukemia. We further reasoned that if this were true, if we removed the pituitary gland from the baby rat shortly after giving the Gross virus, the rat should not develop leukemia, while the rats that had a sham operation should develop leukemia as always.

I made contact with a faculty member over at Tulane University who agreed to teach me how to remove the pituitary gland in a rat. When I arrived with the proper-aged rats in tow, he greeted me with, "You are too old. If you will bring me a seventeen-year-old girl, I can teach her to remove pituitary glands and she will never miss. You are old enough that you won't feel the changes in the route of the needle as it passes into the pituitary fossa (small dip in the floor of the skull where the pituitary gland is located)."

I told him that I didn't have a seventeen-year-old girl at my beck and call, so it was going to have to be me. We gave the rat a little ether, and took a 20 cc syringe containing a little saline and a number eighteen gauge needle, entered it into the rat's ear canal, through the ear drum and into the pituitary fossa. I'll admit that I could not always feel that little dip, but it was a good feeling to pull gently and see the rat's pituitary move into the saline in my syringe. The ones that I missed were our control subjects; that is, they had exactly the same procedure done, but the pituitary gland remained intact. To make a long story short, the rats that had their pituitary gland removed did not grow because they didn't have any growth hormone. Likewise, their T cells didn't start growing and there was no leukemia.

We had proved that acute lymphoblastic leukemia was a hormonal malignancy under the control of the rat's pituitary gland. The next step was to see what caused the continued manufacture of T cells in the thymus of apparently normal humans after a sudden temporary condition called for the manufacture of large numbers of T cells. In other words, some acute condition made a sudden call for large numbers of T cells, but then the thymus gland didn't stop making them even though there was no obvious need for more T cells. The thermostat had to be broken.

Things were percolating along very nicely. However, I was raised during the Great Depression, and I had the same mindset of so many of who were. People who lived through the Great Depression were always looking on the dark side of everything. As my mother used to say, "Things are going too good, something bad is bound to happen." That was certainly true in this case.

Dean Bob Bucher called a meeting of his inner council one day to tell us that the president of the university had confiscated (his word) medical school earned money to make his overall school budget balance. Money that was made through the hospital fees, faculty fees, etc., had accumulated to several hundreds of thousands of dollars that were, according to Bob's recruitment agreement, money that could be used solely to further programs of the medical school. However, everyone apparently knew that the president never let a thing like an agreement stand in his way of doing what he wanted to do. He was the epitome of the Peter Principle when he became a college president after being fired for incompetence by University of Alabama President Dr. Frank Rose when he was director of the University of Alabama extension service in Mobile. He would stride into a room to attend a meeting with all the airs of a caliph. One would expect to see a little black boy in a turban, with a huge feather-fan trailing along behind. Yet when he was around South Alabama Board of Trustee's members, he was an absolute mewing sycophant.

Bob wouldn't back down on this, and a battle actually raged over this money. It became a matter of honor for Bob, and the end result was that he resigned as dean. This was a terrible blow for the school. He switched over to being a surgeon again in the surgery department. I happened to run into him after his first day back in the operating room as an assistant surgeon. I asked him if he found a lot of changes since the last time he had been in the operating room. He answered, "No, not really. I was disappointed to find how little it had changed." Ultimately, he set up a clinic on Dauphin Island which is one of the barrier islands that separates the Gulf of Mexico from the southern Alabama coastline. He practiced there until he died.

This was a blow for the rest of us, as we really liked this concept of close involvement with the practicing physician community. Little did we realize how this was going to change in the future operations.

Ray had an idea that the Leukemia Society might want to sponsor a yearly lecture series at South Alabama. This was not proposed to be a raunchy little affair, but a black-tie event with the absolute top people in the field invited to give one of the proposed yearly events. I spoke with the local representative of the Society and he became very excited about that possibility. He contacted the powers that be in the Society, and they agreed to fund our initial lecture. We decided to invite Dr. Ludwig Gross as the first lecturer, and he accepted our invitation. It was held in the medical school auditorium on the main campus as a black-tie, very formal lecture. Bob Bucher was still dean at the time, and he did a superb job as host of the event. Dr. Gross did not disappoint us with his erudite recounting of the earlier work of virology and malignancies, and his ideas of what the future held in this field. The auditorium was full; the lecture was greatly appreciated, as noted by the ovation Dr. Gross got at the end of his lecture. The Leukemia Society officials liked it well enough to pledge to support the next in the series the following year.

Ray and I continued our search for the trigger that set off the over-stimulation of T cells that leads to acute lymphocytic leukemia. We decided that we would attend the International Conference of Cancer in Florence, Italy, so as to talk with other people who were working along the same lines. We particularly wanted to talk with an investigator at the University of Paris who was using live BCG vaccine to stimulate normal T cell production during clinical remission of the disease, as a method to prevent a relapse. This vaccine was used extensively in earlier years in an attempt to prevent tuberculosis. Ray, Nancy and I took off for Florence, Italy, to attend the international conference. We found our Frenchman, who invited us to visit him at his laboratory after the conference. We spent the rest of the week attending various paper presentations and seeing the sites. Nancy, for some reason, chose to boycott the papers and concentrated on sightseeing.

We were actually staying at a small hotel in a small town outside of Florence. It supposedly was the town where Pinocchio was originated, but I have forgotten the name of it. We were wandering around the village one day when we came upon a small outdoor bazaar. We found a blue shirt that we thought we would buy as a present for Paul. When we told the merchant that we wanted to buy it, he became agitated and didn't want to let us buy it. He didn't speak any English and I didn't speak any Italian, so we did have a failure to communicate. Finally, through the typical Italian arm waving, I could see that he thought I was buying the shirt for myself. I thought and thought about what was the word for child, and suddenly "bambino" came into my head. I said, "For bambino."

With that, he got this huge, toothy grin beaming out from under a big, bushy mustache, and he said, "Ahh, Bambino." He kept repeating it over and over while he put the shirt in a paper bag. He was truly a relieved soul.

We finished our week in Florence and were getting ready to catch a train to Milan. I was thinking back over the huge number of sights we had seen over the past week. I remembered the green granite cathedral with its famous wooden and iron doors in the center of town. I recalled how people would chatter away while looking at all the wonderful artwork, even though church services were being held in many of the naves in the building. In contrast, when we walked two or three blocks down the street to the building where Michelangelo's *David* is kept, everyone spoke in quiet, muffled whispers.

We boarded our train in the Florence railway station and entered our typical European compartment with its two sets of seats facing each other. After settling in, we looked across the compartment to see our traveling companions. There sat Dr. John Day Peak, a radiologist from Mobile. It continued to be a small world. We pulled out of the station and took a train trip through northern Italy's beautiful mountain country. We arrived in the Milan railway station, which was one of Mussolini's contributions to Italian society. He took great pride in keeping the Italian trains running on time. We detrained, and we began walking toward the station carrying all of our baggage. After walking seemingly miles, we finally arrived at the station. I was told that the station was one of the largest in the world. I believed every word of it.

We saw a few places in Milan, including the fresco *The Last Supper* by Leonardo da Vinci. It was in a small church and occupied the entire wall behind the altar. The ceiling was low, and the lighting was dimmer than I would have liked, but no one asked my opinion. This left it to be less monumental in appearance than I thought it should be. People spoke in whispers there also. We caught a plane flying over the Pyrenees to Paris that day.

We flew into Orly airport and got a cab to our hotel, which was a small three-story building with a Mansard roof sitting in the midst of downtown Paris. The first night we walked a couple of blocks down the street to a recommended restaurant. It was a small, efficient place that had excellent food. We ordered French food: steak. A couple of tables over from where we were seated, several waiters and a wine steward were huddled around a single table. There was much hustle and bustle, and they all seemed to be occupied with a single bottle of wine. Finally, the crowd dispersed and our waiter told us that they were trying to open a bottle of wine that had been bottled one hundred years previously. The cork kept crumbling and they were concerned that a piece of the cork might fall into the wine. See, if they had used screw tops, they wouldn't have had that problem.

The next day, we went sightseeing. We went inside Notre Dame Cathedral, and I agree with the farmer: it sure would hold a lot of hay. My favorite place was the Impressionists' museum. I have always liked those paintings very much, and we spent most of the day there. We were driving down the boulevard, and the Eiffel Tower was just ahead. Ray said, "You know, we ought to hire the man who convinced people that the Eiffel Tower is pretty. We could use somebody like that to sell University of South Alabama."

The next day, Ray and I caught the Metro out to the University of Paris. We had a very nice visit (fortunately, he was fluent in English), and we came away with an agreement to use his BCG vaccine on some our patients in clinical remission. We had to go through all sorts of legal machinations, but eventually we started getting shipments of live BCG vaccine from Paris. We carried this on for a long time but could not demonstrate any difference in the BCG patients and the controls.

Along about this time, when Paul was at Georgia Tech and John was a senior in high school, Nancy and I decided to call it quits. It was an emotionally traumatic time for everyone. Both families were greatly upset in this ending that has become so common in modern marriages. I am sure that no one was as upset as the boys. We were very close in those days, and the distance between us has broadened since. This has been a source of quiet despair for me. I moved to an apartment and purchased a condemned house in the Oakleigh Garden District. It had a lot wrong with it, and it was tied up in a family estate with six different family members, one of whom was in a psychiatric hospital. One of the family members happened to be one of our accountants for Children's Medical Group, and he pushed the thing through his family. I paid the princely price of five thousand dollars for the house and lot. Now the fun and games of old home restoration were about to begin.

During this time my mother became ill. She had suffered with rheumatoid arthritis for several years, but this was worse. A diagnosis of lymphoblastoma was made, and chemotherapy was started with the faint hope that it might help. It didn't, and she died the night before hurricane Frederick struck. I lost a very supportive person in my life with that death.

Finally, a new dean was appointed for the medical school. He was a young fellow who had no clue about the duties of a dean. There was no leadership there at all; people were operating on the hope that he would just not get in the way. It was a terrible time to be without leadership: bad habits quickly become established in such situations, and it is extremely difficult for the next dean to exorcise them.

It suddenly was time for the second Leukemia Society Lectureship. This time we asked Bob Good to give the lecture, and he agreed to come. He flew down from New York, as he now was the head of research at Sloan Kettering Institute. He spent two or three days with us, recalling old times. Ray took him fishing on Turkey Creek, which is off Fish River in Baldwin County. This was in cold weather, so they were trolling for anything that might happen along. Suddenly Bob got a strike, and when he set the hook the fish didn't move at all. At first they thought that he might have hung a sunken log, but then the line began to move nonchalantly upstream. Whatever it was, it didn't seem to be even annoyed by having a hook stuck in his mouth. They fought him for around ninety minutes and he never surfaced. In fact, he was a lot more in charge of the situation than Bob was. Whenever he tired of the game, he broke the line. In cold weather, alligator gars stay in Turkey Creek until springtime warms the waters in shallower places. We surmised that he hooked one of those big devils. He was as excited as a little kid and was still talking about it when he got on the plane to leave.

Bob had press conferences and was shown around the school. Part of this itinerary was a visit with the university president. The meeting didn't last too long, but Bob came out shaking his head in bewilderment. "That guy is crazy as a loon" is the only comment he made. We all knew what he was talking about.

Bob gave one of his patented speeches for this occasion–starting slow to explain the basics, and then soaring off into scientific wonderland. He ended the lecture, "In future years, we will look back upon irradiation as a treatment for malignancy the same way we now look at the old practice of putting fuming nitric acid on dog bites to prevent rabies." After the lecture we met with the Leukemia Society representative, and he broke the bad news to us. We had been too successful, and other schools were complaining that we had a lectureship and they didn't. I had been down this path before, and I realized we had lost our funding. There was no hope that the school would bail us out, and they didn't. The lectureship died that night.

It was not long after that everyone agreed, including the dean, that the dean's job needed someone more experienced in it. A search committee was set up and the usual procedures for this type of seeking slowly began to turn. After a while we began to have candidates arrive. Some of these were acquaintances of mine and they would drop by for a chat. To the man, they all thought that the president was a dolt and would not be someone for whom they would like to work. Nobody would touch the job with a ten-foot pole. They eventually put the head of internal medicine up as the new dean.

This was the death knell for the original guys, as this fellow had never had an original thought in his life, and like his boss the president, he didn't like all this inclusion of private practitioners in the teaching programs. This all came to pass, and all the other innovative things that Bob Bucher had instigated were stopped. I had written a grant, in a less expansive plan than at Birmingham, for the improvement of charity pediatric patients' medical and surgical care. I took it in for the dean's signature, and after signing it, he told me that he was looking for someone to be the new chairman of pediatrics who was more in line with his thinking.

He found him, and the guy thought just like the dean. His idea of research was to give some of the cancer patients high doses of vitamin A. He considered himself a nutritionist, but he couldn't pose a rational question that he was trying to answer with this trial or explain why he suggested it. It was not something with which I wanted to be associated. Again, and for the last time, I resigned a professorship of pediatrics. I would later receive a letter from some school committee stating that if I wanted a clinical professor of pediatrics appointment, I would have to apply for it. I didn't bother to answer it. Incidentally, we did get the grant that I requested the dean to sign. I have no idea what happened to it.

Chapter 13

'I Will Practice My Art' — Hey, My Dream Is Happening

Now that I was free from academic entanglements. I realized that I didn't get a great deal accomplished at South Alabama. But from my labor the school did get a well organized department in both clinical and research programs. When the word got out that I was no longer at South Alabama, I began getting phone calls from schools that had chairman vacancies such as Maryland, Johns Hopkins, etc. I simply told them I wasn't interested, after thanking them for thinking of me. I started working on rebuilding my practice.

There was no looking back in regret about what I had not been able to accomplish in my academic years. By now I had accepted the fact that something much higher than I was allowing me to accomplish things wherever I was given the opportunity. Now I had reached that point in life where I had learned to recognize the limits of my capabilities and to move on to what was going to be offered to me next. When this point in one's life is reached and this recognition occurs, it makes the future much more exciting to contemplate. It is never known what new problems are waiting to be met and conquered. Now when bad things do occur, I truly never worry about them; I know that God "has my back."

As I reckoned on all the things that had transpired during the relatively short time that my career in medicine had taken up to this point, it had been a remarkable time. Medicine, since the end of World War II, had made remarkable strides in the development of new sciences, the understanding of the functioning of the body, etc. For instance, great strides have been made in the defining of the immune system so that now it was possible for the transplantation of organs, the treatment of malignancies, and the understanding of the role of immunology in new therapies, auto-immune diseases, etc. Genetics and its role in diseases and other syndromes was just beginning to be explored. The mortality rates of diseases and neonates, as well as the epidemics of diseases, were steadily going down. This was in part due to the growing ability to identify viruses and bacteria, so that vaccines were developed to prevent polio, red measles, German measles, mumps, hemophilus influenza (primary cause of meningitis in children), chicken pox, tetanus, and meningicoccus (main cause of meningitis in teenagers), all of which were done by pediatricians.

Pediatricians are constantly trying to prevent diseases and put themselves out of business. The relief experienced by people with sleep apnea, by the use of CPAP, was developed for treatment of neonates with respiratory distress syndrome. Medicine was easily discerned at this time as being at its zenith. Over the next few years, the peak of medical achievements would begin to flatten and, then, in my opinion, it started to decline. The research began to be directed to instant gratification, such as new methods of surgery, new electronic gadgets, and a spate of buildings devoted to treatment, instead of further basic knowledge of the altered physiology causing a malady. Data in this area of altered physiology leads to the prevention of a disease, so that there is no need for a revolutionary form of therapy. It is an old adage that says it is far easier to prevent a disease than to treat it. In the next few years, I would ruminate on these thoughts as I saw medicine and its professional application of being there for the patient's good begin to slowly decline into a sea of "me first."

While contemplating all of these weighty subjects, I realized that I had more practical problems to solve. The boys and I had been working on my condemned house since I had acquired it. During spare times and weekends, we worked on it together when they weren't tied up with other things. Otherwise, I worked on it alone during the week after work and on weekends. The boys stuck with it but, to say the least, it wasn't their favorite thing to do. They got the lean out of the house, and it looked straight when we looked at it. I really don't think that I ever thanked them enough when we were working on it steadily. We took the roof off the back of the house and added a small library, bedroom, and full bath up there. I hired some guys that Pap recommended from over in Baldwin County to frame up that added-on part upstairs. They were good, steady workers and framed it up with all the proper bracing put in. A short time after that, I read in the local newspaper they had been arrested for armed robbery and shooting somebody. Nice people my own father recommended! Later, he refused to talk about these articles in the paper; he always had other things to do, or suddenly his hearing got bad.

I had the entire house rewired, and Pap and I put in new plumbing. I knew that trade that Pap insisted I learn would someday pay off. The sewer system in the house was cast-iron pipe, and Pap had enough left from his old business to rework the sewer pipe and add a new bathroom upstairs. It had to be put together with lead joints that were caulked by using a special chisel to seal the lead to the pipe and prevent them from leaking. The electricians, who weren't all that young, were fascinated by my doing this. They did more watching of me caulk joints than putting in my new wiring.

By now, Paul had transferred to Vanderbilt and John was enrolled at Berry College. I tried to continue the habit of writing them short letters every week. Paul was pretty good about keeping me up to date, but it was a significant occasion when I got a letter from John. I put reminders on the outside of his letters such as if deceased, please notify sender. It didn't help. Both boys did extremely well in school, and I have always been extremely proud of them.

The practice was growing back very well, and it helped that I was known by so many people in medicine. I had a small girl whom we diagnosed as having neuroblastoma, which is a malignancy that was located in her adrenal gland. The parents were apprehensive about having her treated locally, and said they wanted to talk with some other people about where to take her. That was perfectly all right with me; I always made sure that parents were completely satisfied about being treated locally. In a few days they returned, all ready to begin treatment. They were excited that they had talked with someone at Children's in Chicago, and this person knew of me and said they could do no better anywhere else. I smiled, mumbled something about it was good that we could start, but what I didn't tell them was that that fellow was one of my old residents. The girl's therapy went extremely well, and she is still hale and hearty.

About this time, I adopted a daughter, Rhonda, who was one of my leukemia patients. She is now in her forties and doing well. She had a sister, Valerie, who was a middle-school student. We all three lived together in the Texas Street house while I finished renovating it. I had fun redoing that house. Every room's design came from some famous house featured in books of famous homes. I actually made all the intricate molding in my dad's workshop.

After a short time, Valerie began to chafe under all the high standards I insisted we follow. Things like going to church, taking piano lessons, behaving like a lady, etc., were beginning to be an irritant. It was quite an adjustment to get girls rather than boys ready for school. I became very proficient at ironing dresses and blouses, and the girls never had to attend school in uniforms not nicely pressed, if I do say so myself. After all three of us lived together a little longer, Valerie asked me if I would adopt her. I immediately agreed. When we were in the courtroom, the judge asked Valerie if she asked to be adopted, to which she answered, "Yes." The judge looked at me and said, "You must be proud to have a fine young girl want you to adopt her." He had no idea how proud I was. I played father and mother to both girls for a good while. Through those years when I was mother and father to Valerie, we became very close. I had a marvelous daughter who loved her daddy.

Paul graduated from Vanderbilt, with honors, no less. He immediately went to work for IBM and was sent to Boca Raton, Florida. There he met Jan, who became his wife and the mother of his two sons. Soon after their marriage, he was transferred to Austin, Texas, and they bought their first home in Round Rock, Texas.

John graduated from Berry College, also with honors. We had worried about his getting into veterinary school, since there were only nineteen veterinary schools in the United States at that time. John had an excellent record, and one day I said to him, "John, with your record, we wouldn't have any difficulty getting you into medical school." He looked at me as if I had suddenly lost my mind and said, "I don't want to go to a medical school, I want to go to veterinary school." That ended that not so bright idea, and later he was accepted at Auburn's School of Veterinary Medicine. He did a veterinary surgery residency after graduation. Later he would meet and marry Angela Gretch, also a veterinary student, and they have a thriving practice and five children.

I was seeing patients one afternoon when a lady brought her

adopted son to see me. I had taken care of both of her children since their adoptions. In fact, I had checked both of them for the bureau for Catholic Charities as newborns. Children's Medical Group took care of all the bureau's newborns free of charge, since Pete Bertucci was a strong Catholic. Harrison, the son, had a rash due to fire ant bites. The mother, Betty, lived in the same neighborhood as my renovated home, and she asked me to stop by some evening for a drink. I stopped by that afternoon, but as usual she was taking an afternoon nap. She later invited me to dinner along with some neighborhood people, and, as they say, the rest is history. I chased her until she caught me.

Betty and I were married October 22, 1983—twenty-six years ago. It was the best thing that ever happened to me. We all moved into Betty's house on Selma Street, two newlyweds and four teenage children, Valerie, Rhonda, Harrison and Abigail. Hollywood probably could make a very funny movie about that first year. The kids sort of accepted each other, but it was a grudging acceptance. Rhonda was in the ninth grade and going to a Catholic school. She was having trouble learning it all, and she and I would spend two or more hours every night just completing her homework. I'm glad to say that she passed with flying colors. The amount of food consumed in that household was stupendous. There would be enough to feed an army, and it would all disappear in just a moment. We would come home in the afternoon from work and every light in the house would be on, and the stereo would be blaring so loudly that it seemed as though the walls pulsated to the beat. When they realized that one of us was home, the sound would be immediately lowered and lights began to be cut off.

The first Christmas, Betty wanted to have the family over for a dinner. Unfortunately, a record cold wave came through at the same time. We had several days with temperatures being around zero, which is not supposed to happen in Mobile. All the plumbing was frozen, including the drain pipes. The dining room at that time was just below one of the upstairs baths. We began dinner, which had been magnificently prepared by Betty under very adverse circumstances (no running water, dishwater thrown out the back door because the drains were frozen), when suddenly there came a drip, drip, drip from the ceiling next to the light fixture. It ended in short fashion, and we simply didn't worry about it too much. It was the last time that we used all the fireplaces in the house, and after dinner John fell asleep on the floor, with his head almost on the hearth of a glowing coal fire. I worried about him baking his brain or something.

The next day we all went to work, and when Betty got home that afternoon she could hear what she described as "Niagara Falls." She went into the kitchen, where a sink pipe was spewing water. As she was looking at this, she saw some type of movement in the dining room. She looked and saw a steady stream of water issuing forth from the ceiling next to the chandelier. She called me at the office, and I, in turn, called Paul and John. They came running, along with Jan, Paul's wife. They got to the house before I did and helped Betty move the dining table out of the deluge. By the time I arrived, water was flowing more freely, and we got the chandelier down just seconds before the ceiling collapsed. Then gallons on top of gallons of water came cascading down into the dining room.

The tub faucets had been inadvertently left on before the pipes froze. The water pipes had thawed enough to allow water to run into the bathtub, but the drain was still frozen. After filling the tub the water had to go somewhere, so it overflowed into the dining room below. It's funny now, but there was very little humor derived from it at the time. One of my priorities with the house became insulating water pipes and closing the underpinning of the house on the north side. We also had another positive thing from it: the insurance company paid for everything to be fixed. This included the insulation of the area which was not present before the catastrophic event.

My referral practice grew by leaps and bounds, and I was seeing as many odd diseases in patients as I did when I was a departmental chairman. I got a referral of a baby with a hemangioma (massive numbers of blood vessels massed together in the skin) on her entire right cheek. These people were from South Carolina, and I don't remember how I wound up seeing them here in Mobile. Well, these types of hemangiomas disappear over time, but it looks horrible to the poor patients. I explained that it would disappear in time, but I would find out who was the best person in South Carolina to follow the child's progress. I picked up the phone and called the chairman of pediatrics at the University of South Carolina School of Medicine. We chatted and joked for a few minutes, and he gave us the name of a pediatric dermatologist to follow the child. They were greatly impressed, but I didn't tell them that the guy was my chief resident one year at Alabama and served his fellowship in infectious disease with Hugh Dillon.

And it came to pass that Jan's time came to deliver Paul's and her firstborn son, Steven. They were living in Round Rock, Texas, a suburb of Austin, at this time. We had prepared for this moment by my building a cradle that was a duplicate of the Steven Crooms' family cradle. We had ideas that this would be the Bentley family cradle, but that didn't work out. When I finished it, Valerie and I were going to drive out to Texas with the cradle so it would be in the home after delivery. I went down to U-Haul and rented a trailer to carry the cradle. We drove over to Fairhope to pick it up, but when we tried—shades of Miss Emma Lamb— the cradle was too big for the door. I tried to replace the trailer in Fairhope and Spanish Fort, but no one had the size I needed. I had to drive all the way back to Mobile, swap trailers, drive back to the Eastern Shore, and finally get the cradle into a trailer.

My dad didn't help my mood any by laughing that I had rented a trailer with too small a door. We finally started out to Texas around three-thirty in the afternoon. We spent the night just over the Texas state line and drove on to Round Rock the next day. We arrived about one o'clock in the afternoon, unloaded the trailer, and turned it in to the dealership. We only got to stay about an hour before we had to start back, which was irritating to Paul that we had such a short stay. However, I had to be home the following day. We stopped at a Mexican restaurant in Houston so Valerie could have some real Tex-Mex food. Her appetite did it justice.

When Steven was about five or six months old, Betty and I decided that we would spend our short vacation going out to see the new grandson and then do a little sightseeing on the way back. On the drive out there, Betty informed me that a friend of ours told her that I was listed in a book she had looked at in her doctor's office. She said that it was something about my being one of the one thousand best physicians in the United States. I made a mental note of it, but I wasn't too impressed. How could anybody presume to select the best one thousand doctors in the United States?

We drove on to Round Rock, and I got to meet my new grandson. He was a very wise and precocious young lad, and he was very glad to see his granddaddy. I'm pretty sure that he went into a state of depression when I left.

On the way back home, I convinced Betty that we should go home via Mountain Home, Arkansas, and let me introduce her to rainbow trout fishing on the White River. I could tell that she was not overjoyed with this prospect, but gamely, she smiled and said something like, "It sounds like it might be fun." We checked into a motel, and the next morning drove out to the boat-renting place on the White River. Stupidly, in an effort to save money, I decided we did not need to hire a guide. I was sure that I had been there enough times that I could put us right on the trout. We were using canned yellow corn for bait, which Betty immediately began to ridicule. We started off downstream and didn't even smell a rainbow trout. After a while, I decided that we should head back to the dock.

It was then that I noticed that the water level had lowered noticeably. They had closed the water gates on the dam. On the return voyage, rocks that had been far underwater on the way down river were now shearing propeller pins with great regularity. We finally came upon a large submerged rock that could not be seen, and we, unfortunately, wedged the boat firmly into one of its crevices. Betty reluctantly stepped overboard into the truly icy water and began tugging. Suddenly the boat came off the rock and released all resistance to Betty's pulling on the boat. Betty fell straight backward and was immersed in ice water up to her neck. In addition, she hit the rocks on the bottom of the river and badly bruised her tailbone.

She climbed back in the boat, cursing under her breath, but not so softly that I couldn't hear every word. She taught me some new words, which she told me later she had learned from Dr. Champ Lyons in the operating room. We finally got back to the dock, returned the boat, and headed back to the motel with the heater on high. We had rainbow trout that night for dinner in the motel's dining room. It was our only glimpse of rainbow trout for the entire trip. The next morning we left Arkansas, drove to Natchez, Mississippi, and toured old antebellum homes for the rest of the trip. While we were up in the Ozark Mountains of Arkansas, Betty bought a very small churn at a pottery. When we got home, we found it leaked.

Paul continued to work in Texas, and according to company protocol, he was moved to Birmingham to obtain sales experience, as I understood it. Shortly after moving, the virus that plagued us with moves struck them also, and Jan became pregnant. Keith was born when Steven was about eighteen or nineteen months old. Now Paul and Jan were the proud parents of two fine boys. We became very close with Jan, and she enjoyed coming down to Mobile and staying for a few days at a time. Jan and Betty became very close, and they became more like sisters than mother-in-law and daughter-in-law.

They eventually moved again to Irondale, a suburb of Birmingham, where they had a great deal more room for outside playing. Around the time that Keith was in the first grade and Steven was in the third grade, Paul called one day after dark. He said that Jan was having bad pains in the right upper abdomen. After questioning him about the pain a little more, I told him that it sounded like liver pain and she should see someone that night. It turned out to be colon cancer, with a lot of involvement of the liver. Of course they tried everything, but the prognosis was bad. She suddenly started having trouble breathing one day and Paul called us. Nancy was already there.

By the time we arrived, Jan had gotten a lot worse. She was having very difficult breathing. Betty sat down beside her, held her hand, and began talking quietly into her ear. When Betty started talking, Jan seemed to relax and quit fighting the inevitable end. She died that night, and the last thing that we did when we were getting ready to go back to Mobile for the funeral was to go by the funeral home. Betty got out of the car, went in by herself, and made sure that everything was all right with Jan's body as Jan had requested before she died. This was a very catastrophic time for all of us, and try as we might, we couldn't help Paul too much with the boys. He later found and married Jennifer, who had three children of her own. They eventually built a home in Trussville, Alabama, where they live now.

Harrison finished high school and joined the Marines. It was a life for which he was truly meant. After finishing his first four-year stint, he tried being in the New Orleans Police Department. This was a place that was exceeded only by Cook County, Illinois, for its corruption. After a short spread of time trying his hand at heavy construction, he returned to his true home, the United States Marine Corps, as a sergeant. He has served in Bosnia and was one of the team that rescued Scott O'Grady. He had two tours in Iraq, and we all hope (including his young daughter Hannah), his active-duty days are over.

Abigail finished high school, and she decided to attend Montevallo University. This was a total disaster as she had not reached the emotional maturity needed for college life. She returned home and worked at a variety of jobs before she met and married

Frank Parrish. Frank joined the Air Force and received his college degree in accounting while still in the service. While stationed in California, Abigail became pregnant and delivered her first son, Frank Roland Parrish, IV, whom we all call Roland.

About five years later, while living in San Antonio, Texas, Abigail brought forth her second son, the whirling dervish Will. There have been no dull times associated with Will since he was born. Abigail would go on to graduate from the University of Texas-San Antonio with a degree in elementary education. She has become an excellent kindergarten teacher in whom we all take great pride. They live in the Houston, Texas, area, where Frank is currently a manager with the large accounting firm Ernst and Young.

The entire time I practiced pediatrics after leaving academic medicine, I received phone calls from former students or other physicians asking for my ideas on one of their patients, etc. Sometimes it would be old acquaintances, such as Willard Blankenship calling from the University of California-Davis to ask me to consider coming to look at the chairmanship of pediatrics where he was a faculty member. I essentially told him that I had all that kind of experience that I needed. He was really disappointed, reminding me of all the things we had done at Alabama to get the department going. Later, one of my former residents called from Tennessee wanting the same thing. I gave him the same answer, and he, too, was sorely disappointed.

So it was not a surprising thing when I got a call from one my former students, Larry Thead, who had a family practice in Demopolis, Alabama. He called often for advice, so I was not surprised to hear from him. This time it was different. He began to relate a story about a little girl named Victoria, who was afflicted with congenital psoriasis. Psoriasis is a skin disease characterized by red, scaly rash that leads to bleeding of the rash when it is scratched, and it can occur anywhere there is skin. It has been shown to be one of the autoimmune diseases where the patient exhibits antibodies against his or her own skin. It is a chronic illness without a cure or much relief.

This little girl was, at that time, six years old and had suffered with the malady since infancy. Larry said that she had this scaly red unsightly rash all over her, and even her ear canals were clogged, so that he couldn't see the eardrums. He explained to the mother that this needed to be treated by a competent dermatologist, and he needed to refer her to the medical center in Birmingham. That is when he said the mother gave him a lesson in medical economics. She said, "Doctor, if you send me to Birmingham, I will have to hire someone to carry me. Then when I see the doctor up there, I will have to pay him. When I get back home after getting a prescription, I won't have the money to buy the medicine. You will just have to find something to treat her with."

Larry said that he phoned his pharmacy friend and asked him, "What are they using nowadays to treat psoriasis?" His friend answered that they were using fluorinated cortisone, but the parents couldn't afford that. Larry told him, "If that comes in generic, we'll use it. I need to put a little salicylate in there to take the scales off, and a little coal tar to just help clear all the debris. Now what can we add from over the counter drugs that has salicylate in it? Aspercreme; we'll add some Aspercreme to it."

They worked out the percentages and it was filled. In Demopolis, they do prescriptions differently than anywhere else that I know. The doctor calls in the prescription, it is filled, and then it is delivered to the doctor's office. The physician then hands the drugs to the patient and goes over the instructions of its use. Larry said that the mother should put it on Victoria's rash daily and call him in two weeks. In the meantime, he intended to find an "angel" to pay for her trip to Birmingham and buy the medicine. She called back in two weeks as requested, and she told Larry that it looked like she was better. Larry responded, "Yes, yes. Just keep putting on her medicine and check with me in another two weeks." When she returned, he called me. "Dr. Bentley, she's completely cleared."

This was indeed an amazing discovery. Since that time, Larry has treated innumerable so-called autoimmune diseases. John and Angela helped us to look into the physiology of the entire aspect by using "Victoria's Mixture" on immune problems in dogs. Flea allergy is a very common entity in dogs, where the bites of fleas cause dogs to shed the hair on their back and rear end. Angela and John had a little over twenty dogs they had amassed by deciding to keep the dogs rather than euthanize the animals when they were brought in by their owners. All had some type of physical malformation, and some had obvious skin allergy to flea bites. Checking animals for allergy to fleas showed a hypersensitivity to fleas on intramural injections in all the dogs. Simply putting the mixture daily on a spot of skin where the dog cannot lick it off caused complete reversal of the allergy, as measured by skin testing. Hair quickly regrew with complete healing of the skin in a few weeks.

Red mange in dogs is caused by a mite that gets in the skin of the animal, causing sores. Regular mange is treated by dipping the animal in a solution, thus killing the mite. A healthy immune system then prevents a recurrence. In red mange, the dog has a deficiency in its production of T cell lymphocytes, so it cannot be mobilized to fight off a recurrence of the mites. With such an impaired immune system, the skin lesions become chronic and eventually fatal. However, by putting a small amount of our mixture on a mite-infested dog where it cannot be licked off, such as in an ear, the immune system does develop properly functioning T cells and the immune system becomes effective in killing the invading skin mites.

Around this same time, immunologists began looking at autoimmune diseases in a different way. In the human body, none of the cells live the lifetime of that body. New cells are constantly being made to replace the ones which have become worn out and inefficient. There is an antibody normally made in the body for each type of cell. These antibodies are very specific for a certain cell so that there is no crossover of cell destruction, and when they are needed to do a little tidying up of some old cells, they attack those cells until something tells them to stop. Our previous analogy of a thermostat applies here. Unless something stops the production of a normal janitorial antibody intended for the clearing of old cells of a very specific type, the antibody continues to be made and continues to destroy those same type, but now they are young, healthy cells.

We know from the red mange dogs that our mixture causes normal T cells to be made that cause the production of B cells to produce a competent antibody against mange mites. We know that since each antibody is made specifically against a single antigen, then the control of "normal" antibodies against someone's own cells are under the control of T cells to either be made or cease being made. Since "Victoria's Mixture" stimulates T cell production, as in the dogs with red mange, it is doing the same thing in people with autoimmune diseases such as psoriasis, atopic eczema, Cohn's disease, lupus erythematosis, etc. We have hundreds of examples of these diseases being completely cured or brought under control. We also had zero luck getting anyone to pay attention to a family physician who may have the answer to many of the diseases of the world. I have spoken to many of my immunology friends, and they all answer, "Yeah, yeah." University physicians develop an attitude about practicing physicians so they secretly think these "family docs" are dolts and shouldn't be thinking about such weighty matters. It is far above their capabilities; just look at their empty bibliographies. This is too important a discovery to let it be unknown to practicing physicians. We are currently preparing to submit our findings for publication, including the control of flea allergy and red mange in dogs. After all, dogs need relief just like humans. Following that, we plan an article on clearing atopic eczema, then one on our experiences of clearing more psoriasis patients, Crohn's disease, etc., so other patients can have complete relief from these autoimmune diseases.

Valerie finished the first two years of college and decided to get married. After she married, Valerie continued school and did very well. She said that she took school a lot more seriously when she paid for it rather than me. She graduated from the University of South Alabama with a degree in accounting and formed her own accounting business after becoming a CPA. She had my first girl grandchild, Rebecca, who would later give me my first great-grandchild, Mark. He has the same red hair as his grandmother, along with the same temper that goes with it.

After about fifteen years of being solely in private practice, I began to discern a change in the practice of medicine. Suddenly, physicians were becoming more involved with owning boats, expensive cars, and large fancy houses and offering less physician time per patient. It was not hard to also discern a change in peoples' attitudes toward physicians as these physicians' behavior patterns became more common. People were feeling as if the physicians who were behaving in this manner were more interested in what money could be made rather than their patients. A lot of these physicians developed the attitude of "fighting their practice," where the physicians were resenting the intrusion of patients on their time.

Suddenly, the occurrence of medical malpractice suits began to appear on the trial dockets in the county court houses. It was not difficult to anticipate that, with the decreased respect that physicians were now regarded by their patients, juries of their local peers were not going to shield them from malpractice suits. It was just a trickle at first, and I spoke with a practicing attorney who was a friend of mine about my concern over these suits. He told me that I shouldn't worry too much about that because medical malpractice suits were very uncommon in Alabama. Several years later, during the "blood in the water" feeding frenzy of trial lawyers, the magazine *Medical Economics* had a long article naming the three worst places to practice medicine in the United States based on the awards given by juries. These were listed as Long Island, New York; Cook County (Chicago), Illinois; and Mobile, Alabama. So much for using the past to predict the future.

During this time, the insurance company where most Alabama physicians purchased their medical malpractice announced that it would longer write malpractice policies in Alabama. There were no other insurance companies eager to take up this glut of uninsured physicians. Most of these physicians eventually bought stock in a small Alabama insurance company, and it was changed into a medical malpractice insurance company. Those were troublesome times without any malpractice coverage. Physicians began to divest themselves of actual ownership of homes, cars, boats, real estate, etc. In effect we physicians owned nothing and other members of the family were actual owners. This prevented our private possessions from being taken if a judgment for a sum of money exceeded our insurance coverage.

During these unsettling times, another common thing began happening that was exceedingly irritating to all physicians. About every two or three weeks, it was not uncommon for one of the members of our group to receive a letter from some trial lawyer stating that so and so had retained them to pursue litigation against the physician for some contrived complaint. However, if one of us would send a sum of ten, twenty, or thirty thousand dollars as a settlement, then the case would need to go no further. No one ever responded personally to the letter, and they were just sent on to the insurance company. We never heard from the lawyer anymore. It became so consistent that the office business manager just sent them to the insurance company without discussion. I always looked at it as attempted extortion. After a few years, this practice abated somewhat, along with the frequency of malpractice suits. For several years until my retirement, I looked in the morning paper at the courthouse records for the preceding day to see if I or some other physician was being sued. Slowly the number of medical malpractice suits became less frequent, but never ceased. There are still enough around so that physicians constantly look over their shoulders for the trial lawyer. It makes for an unhappy workplace. The next victims were the nursing homes with alleged patient neglect. Now, the most common thing is the pharmaceutical business. One sees an endless procession of TV ads proclaiming various diseases that apparently have a court settlement for anyone harmed by a certain illness caused by exposure to some substance or drug causing mesothelioma or other maladies. The ads proclaim that you may be eligible for a large cash award. The novel *The Chamber* by John Gresham explains this tactic fully. If one of these lawyers has some patients lined up already, and if he or she can add more up to say, one hundred clients by these large nets trolling through the TV sets, and then if they get several thousands of dollars as their fee from each one of the one hundred clients, this begins to run into serious money. I am sure that you have heard the lament of the old politician: "A billion here, a billion there, and pretty soon you are into serious money."

During these times, a trial was held in Mobile which was going to greatly affect the cost of medical care. It didn't attract any attention, and I became aware of it because one of the defense lawyers asked me to unofficially look over the accusations listed in the complaint against a drug manufacturer who manufactured polio oral vaccine. This was an infant who received oral Sabin polio vaccine as part of her routine care by her physician. Shortly thereafter, she developed paralysis of one of her lower extremities. This was immediately seized upon as a child with poliomyelitis caused by her routine oral polio vaccine. The mother, of course, testified that she never would have allowed the child to take the vaccine if she had known that there was any possibility of it causing her child to develop poliomyelitis. To complicate the matter, the father was a seaman who had returned home from a trip to the Orient, and the child had demonstrated the symptoms shortly after his return. All the "experts" had testified that this was an obvious case of poliomyelitis evidently caused by her immunization. Further strengthening their conclusion was the finding of large quantities of the type of polio vaccine virus given in the child's stools. Of course, that is exactly what is supposed to happen. One of the values of oral vaccine over injected vaccine is that it does continue to grow in the bowel and "contaminate" the entire household and playmates, thus producing "herd immunity." This is the reason polio is very seldom seen now, and any outbreak can quickly be brought under control by oral vaccination. There are also other viral infections that cause clinical signs and symptoms identical to what is seen in poliomyelitis. There was no way to scientifically deny the assumed diagnosis because other causative viruses could no longer be demonstrable at this stage of the illness. The Mobile jury lived up to its reputation and ruled for the plaintiff. At the time, there were only two companies producing polio vaccine. Soon after having to pay the enormous settlement, the polio vaccine manufacturer made the decision to stop this phase of its business. This left only one company providing polio vaccine. Suddenly there was a shortage of polio vaccine and the price tripled owing to the cost of malpractice insurance for the remaining company. Similar trials were held with DPT (diphtheria, pertussis, and tetanus) vaccines with similar results. Whereas one was able to give all these immunizations for about ten dollars, now they were costing thirty-five to forty dollars. The cost of medical care increased again.

In my way, I was able to offer some relief in the doctor's desires for costly cars. I bought a used small-size Ford pickup truck as my personal vehicle. It rode well and was a great deal more practical for hauling, etc., than a very expensive Lexus Runabout. It was not long before trucks were a common sight in the doctor's parking lots. Of course, most of these trucks were virtual behemoths that dwarfed my little Ford.

About this time, HMO's (Health Management Organizations) began to make their presence known. Suddenly we were deluged with all types of these organizations being formed and wanting us to join their ranks, to be part of their collection of physicians to care for the children enrolled in their health care systems. We finally accepted one offer and began to see their patients on a fixed-rate basis per visit. At first, everything went well, but then one day I was examining a newborn baby who was just barely twenty-four hours old. The HMO just allowed one day post-delivery for hospitalization of both the mother and the child. However, the baby was already jaundiced, and it was going to require some time under the bili-light for another day or so in order to prevent possible brain damage from elevated bilirubin blood levels.

Very innocently, I put in a call to the HMO and talked with some management person who was supposedly a nurse. I explained to her the situation and the fact that the child needed to be kept for a time to treat the hyperbilirubinemia and to be certain serum bilirubin levels did not get too high. She asked me what the level was and I told her. She apparently looked at some chart she had and told me that that was one mgm percent too low to qualify for the baby being kept in the hospital. I said very calmly, "You do understand that I am standing here looking at this baby, and you are somewhere else telling me that this baby has to be discharged from the hospital against my clinical judgment?"

She said impertinently, "Yes, we will not pay for the child's hospitalization if you do not discharge the child with its mother."

I calmly replied, "You do realize that the child will just need to be readmitted?"

She said unbelievably, "Well, that will be all right, if that is necessary, but now she must be discharged." I discovered that bureaucrats are the same in the business world as they are in the government, and it makes no difference if one is talking with a medical professional or a pointy-headed government bureaucrat. I had learned to go around this type of bureaucracy before. I discharged the child and then immediately readmitted her to the hospital for her therapy. No one said a word to me about it.

Later I began to ruminate on this happening, and it struck me that this HMO was putting up obstacles to our practicing proper pediatrics. We dropped our participation in that HMO shortly thereafter. This represents the introduction of a third party between the physician and the patient to interfere solely on a business basis. It would have been much better to have a professional discussion than to have a unilateral decision based on an arbitrary chart. At the time of my retirement these types of interferences were becoming more frequent, and they frequently tied up one or two of our office personnel for long periods of time. This increased our cost of taking care of such patients.

Earlier in my private practice years, the services of specially trained registered nurses as PAs (physician assistants) began to be used by practicing physicians to lighten the workload of the physician, both in their offices and in making hospital rounds. These individuals were registered nurses who were given more training so that they could screen patients for acute problems entering the office, make hospital rounds with the physician, and see that everything that needed to be done with a patient was carried out. They made themselves indispensable in the everyday running of a practice, but as with all good things, they went further than was originally intended.

For example, some physicians who didn't want to make hospital rounds were sending their PAs to make unsupervised house rounds. I am sure that they had a great deal of trust in their PA's abilities, but making rounds on patients requires more knowledge to evaluate a patient's clinical status than can be taught in a PA's added education. I had an experience that was used to tighten the reins on overexpansion of a PA's duties.

I received a request from a physician for me to see a six-year-old boy who had been hospitalized for several days with fever and some cough. I saw the child that afternoon on evening hospital rounds and found him to be more sickly in his appearance than I was expecting to see. It turned out that he had not been seen by his physician since he had been admitted to the hospital, but he had been seen daily only by his PA. He was having some pain in his abdominal area, and on listening to his lungs, I could hear abnormal sounds in his right lower lung. A mass could be felt in his left upper abdomen, and after a few tests I determined that he had a malignancy (neuroblastoma) that had already metastasized to his lung.

We treated him with the appropriate drugs, and he began to slowly improve clinically. We were never able to get ahead of the tumor, however, in spite of treating with the latest experimental drugs. One day, the time came when I had to sit down with the child's parents to discuss the deteriorating situation. I explained to them that we had done about everything that we could do. There were some other experimental drugs that we could try, but they were very toxic, which would make him sicker, and they had really not shown to be that effective. We decided that we would not do anything but would just keep him comfortable until the end.

It was not too long before he was not physically able to return to the office for checkups, and his family rented a hospital bed and placed it in his room. My nurse, Scotty, and I would go out to the house, about fifteen miles away, biweekly during our lunch recess. One problem was that it was summertime and my truck had no air-conditioning unit. Scotty suffered through several trips, and then she insisted that we travel in her Volvo, which was cool. The boy gradually worsened and the end seemed near. One week, I had something come up that was going to require my being out of town for a weekend. I was going to make arrangements with one of my partners to be on standby in case he took a turn for the worse while I was gone. The parents wanted to use their old physician, however, and with great trepidation I called the fellow. I explained to him that our plan was to do nothing, and if he got a call to come see him, do not do anything, but allow him to quietly die. The boy had gone bad while I was gone. The doctor did come out, but he started IV fluids and some antibiotic. He successfully resuscitated him. Instead of dying peacefully, he lingered and lingered. He became blind and required IV morphine to keep him comfortable. Every time I visited, I silently cursed that quack. The boy mercifully died about six months later in a late afternoon.

That is a classic example of a physician not carrying out his duties to his patient by not seeing him daily while he was hospitalized. If a patient is sick enough to be admitted to a hospital, he or she deserves to be seen by the physician, given a physical examination and a clinical appraisal daily. They certainly shouldn't put the onus of patient care and evaluation on someone who is not educated sufficiently to fulfill that role. It has become an increasingly prevalent practice for physicians to enter a patient's room, never physically touch the patient, discuss the patients progress with the nurse, say to the patient, "Very good, then, I'll see you tomorrow." This is supposed to be hospital rounds. I consider it pathetic.

One morning toward the end of my practicing days, I was busily seeing patients in my office when Sharon, my nurse, entered and in a low voice told me that there was a child in room four that needed to be seen as soon as I was through here. Fortunately, I was almost finished, so I was able to join her quickly. As we walked to the examining room, she filled me in. Apparently, this little girl had been hospitalized for two or three days with what was diagnosed as a mild pneumonia, with some x-ray abnormalities on a chest x-ray. The admitting physician came in that morning and chastised both parents for being "overly protective" of her. She explained that the child was just not that sick and could easily be taken care of at home.

The parents both protested vehemently, but the physician was adamant. The parents were so overwrought by this happening that they called an ENT physician in town who happened to be a personal friend. He instructed the parents to just take their child to our office and to see any of us who would be able to see her. Sharon just happened to be at the front desk when they entered. The parents told their story; Sharon took one look at the child and she said, "Come with me."

When I entered the room both parents were pacing the floor, and the father had the child, who looked to be about four years old. She was draped over the dad's chest with her head on his shoulder;

it was easy to see that she was having difficulty in breathing. Her inspirations were accomplished with obvious difficulty.

I introduced myself and told the father, "Let me listen to her chest." I listened, and there were no breath sounds at all on the left side of her chest. I told them that I needed to readmit her to another hospital and ordered a chest x-ray on admission. In a short while, the radiologist called to tell me that the left lung area was completely opaque, but they could not identify the heart, so they had no way to know whether the opaque left chest was lung, tumor, or a vastly enlarged heart. I immediately called for a pediatric cardiology consult, and he catheterized her heart and injected a small amount of radio-opaque dye. The heart was normal, but the vessels to the left lung were compressed and shoved to the back of the left thorax.

I talked to the father on the phone and told him that his daughter had a tumor filling most of the left chest cavity. I explained that I needed to refer her to St. Jude's Hospital in Memphis, Tennessee, as I would be retiring in two or three years and was not adding any new oncology patients. However, I took care of most of the St. Jude patients during their home visits, etc. He immediately agreed and I called and told them the situation. I was sending her up by air ambulance, and they should have an ambulance to meet the flight. During the flight up she stopped breathing twice, but they were able to start her back without much difficulty. They took her to St. Jude's and placed her on a respirator, and she became well oxygenated. Subsequently, a biopsy revealed a large thymic tumor, and she was treated with the appropriate therapy and recovered.

A few years ago I received a high school graduation announcement; and this year I received an invitation to her graduation from a very fine Catholic college with cum laude honors. She enclosed a photograph, revealing herself to currently be a beautiful, young woman. I wrote her a note expressing my pride in her accomplishment of turning into a beautiful young lady, but also evidently a very smart one. She wrote me back thanking me for the note, and she informed me that she was starting medical school this fall. This time we had a happy ending, but the physician allowed her annoyance with the parents for what she perceived to be over concern to cloud her clinical judgment. She forgot the old admonition that if a mother says a child is acting differently than your perception, it is very prudent to listen to her. She knows the child much better than you.

I was sued only once, and that was by the father of a child who had cyanosis (blue skin color) all of his life. He had been worked up at Harvard, but they had not found the cause. We eventually found that he had shunts of venous blood into the arterial blood just before they became capillaries all over his body, especially in the lungs. There was nothing that could be done for this child, and we got the father enrolled in our weekly meetings of parents of children with incurable illnesses which met in Children's Medical Group's conference room. The time came, the child died, and we thought we had helped the parents to accept the inevitable. It is the duty of every physician to prepare the patient and his or her family to understand the inevitability of the disease process, and to learn to accept and deal with it on an emotional basis. We failed on this one. I was sued because it was said that I didn't do enough to prolong the child's life. It was thrown out of court. I had a lawyer tell me that I shouldn't take it personally. That happens to be the stupidest statement I have ever heard.

I had another brush with the malpractice attorneys one other time. Several years ago, I had a little girl about three years of age referred to me after surgery revealed a neuroblastoma. This had been removed, and we treated her with chemotherapy and irradiation with apparently excellent results. Every person who has treated many children with this tumor knows how unpredictable it can be. It can be very malignant; it can appear hopeless when viewed at surgery, only to have the malignancy simply disappear with no therapy; it can become a benign tumor (ganglioneuroma), or a ganglioneuroma can convert to a neuroblastoma.

This child's father was a professional fisherman, and her mother was seemingly a very nice young lady. We followed her for about two years, and they suddenly moved after her father was arrested for drug smuggling. About ten years to the day from the time I last saw her, she appeared in my office with her mother. Her mother now had tattoos on both lower legs, and this fourteen-year-old girl had an older boy with her, whom the mother introduced as her daughter's "main squeeze." She had been examined out in Texas a few weeks earlier and found to have a mass at the site of her previous tumor. I found that she did have a mass in the same area, and we surmised that it was a benign recurrence. She was referred to a surgeon who removed a benign mass.

Before she went to surgery, we received a request for her

medical records from a trial lawyer, and in a week or two the notice of a malpractice suit being filed was printed in the local newspaper. (I still looked for my name in the list of people being sued every morning.) I knew what had happened: the dates of her last visit were very close to the date she came to us for her last visit. Apparently, no one in the attorney's office had ever noticed that they were ten years apart. The suit was quietly dropped, but this was not published in the local paper. This type of legal harassment was one of the main reasons that I retired from medicine. A lot of my contemporaries did the same. There was no pleasure to be derived from having a new patient if the doctor looked at him or her as a future litigator rather than a new patient needing help.

This surge of malpractice litigation has had a great detrimental effect on the physicians' practice. To begin with, it completely takes away the joy of being a family's physician and taking care of the family's various maladies and traumatic events. When sued, the first thing that is determined is whether the family physician is qualified to handle the problem that the suit is about. The idea is always planted, or the attempt made to show, that the family doctor is doing things that he or she is not qualified to do. Since a medical student has to spend a two-year residency after a year of internship to become a family practitioner, the student might as well spend the same or slightly more time and become a specialist where this sort of treatment is much less frequent.

This attempt to show that you are less competent than a hired gun as an expert witness is a common tactic. I had the experience of this while being questioned during a deposition in a malpractice suit by a hot Miami lawyer. I had differed with the lawyer's expert witness on the handling of a patient by the defendant, a Miami pediatrician. The lawyer asked me in a sarcastic tone why his expert and I disagreed on the patient's care. He then got this supercilious grin on his face, and with sarcasm dripping from his words he asked, "Perhaps he is a better doctor than you."

I replied, "I don't think so; I'm listed as one of the one hundred best doctors in the United States." This caught him completely unawares, and he sputtered and stammered for two minutes before regaining his equanimity. That was the only time I was ever able to use that bit of information in my behalf. I did say it with a grin on my face.

This information had resulted from an earlier experience. During my time in medicine I testified many times as an expert witness. I must say that in no case in which I ever testified did we lose the case. I sort of enjoyed the game of thwarting their parries, trying to cross me up. In preparing my curriculum vitae for the defense lawyer in a case, the lawyer wanted to impress the jurors as much as he could with his expert witness. He told me to put down everything that I had been listed in so that they could use it in comparing their expert witness to me. I remembered the thing about being named what I thought was one of the best one thousand doctors in the United States. When I looked into it, I found that it wasn't one thousand doctors, but one hundred doctors. I really couldn't see how anyone could narrow the quality of medical care to see who the best one hundred were. I filled out my curriculum vitae with, "Listed in Who's Who in America, in Who's Who in the World, in Leaders of the English Speaking World, and listed as one of the one hundred best doctors in the United States." Of course, none of it meant anything to anyone but my mother.

I practiced pediatrics until I was sixty-five years old. I enjoyed it all until the end of my practice. I enjoyed taking care of my patients, but medicine had changed. It had become more of a business instead of a profession. A physician wasn't anyone's doctor anymore; he or she was whoever had an opening in their schedule. Since then, I haven't missed the practice of medicine the way it was carried on the latter years. I recall with fondness funny things that happened while working. I won't bother you with a litany of these, but I will give you two of my favorites. The first involves a distraught mother who brought her young son in to see us one night when Scotty Dixon, my nurse, and I were working the late shift. The mother said tearfully, "He put a rock in his ear. I poured some water in the other ear, but it didn't come out." Even Scotty, the master of tact, had to turn around to stifle a guffaw.

The other involves one of my partners, who shall remain nameless, and this event was told by his nurse of about fifteen or twenty years, who thought it too good not to be shared. It must be understood that when examining a patient, some requests for the patient become a matter of rote. The perpetrator of this tale was examining a child and needed to look at the rectal opening. He turned the child to the face down position, spread the cheeks of the buttocks, looked at the rectal opening, and said, "Say, Ah."

When it came time for Children's Medical Group to find

a replacement for my slot in the physicians' roster, we let the graduating pediatrics residents in surrounding teaching programs, and around the southern United States, know about our need for a new pediatrician. When each applicant was told how we functioned, the number of patients seen and hours worked, the applicants fell by the wayside like dead flies. They finally filled the slot with a pediatrician who was already in practice and knew the hours worked. This trend of wanting an eight-hour-a-day job, five days a week, has just increased—not diminished. I am sad to say that my old practice is not caring for patients with the diligence that we previously required. That is not one of those "now let me tell you how it was when I was a boy" stories.

This lack of willingness to work for the patient, regardless of the number of hours required, is something that has to be instilled by the medical school professors during the formation of a code of ethics of physician behavior. The quality of graduates of our medical schools might be good academically, but their devotion to duty as a caring physician is essentially lacking. This also has to have something to do with the admissions policy to our medical schools. The professional attitude of a great number of today's graduates shows that the admission committee's choices for admission to medical school are far from good. It seems clear to me that the committees seldom, if ever, look at the results of their choices. I do not mean in an academic sense, but in a devotion to patient care sense. Certainly the product that medical schools are admitting and graduating is more inclined toward being a trade where one is paid according to acquired skills rather than a profession where things are done for the public good.

Now it is fashionable for the candidate for admission to medical school to spend a year in some community charity activity. This is not a printed requirement in the published admission requirements, but it is well known to all applicants that this is true. In addition, they should "shadow" a practicing physician to observe the actual practice of medicine and see if they want to emulate him. No one evaluates the physician that they "shadow," to see if that individual is a good doctor who enjoys taking care of his patients, or if he or she is one of the "new physicians" who are the eight-hour-a-day wonders. It doesn't take long for the word to leak out that the school wants this to be done for one to become a viable candidate.

Now it becomes another "under the rug" requirement that

an aspiring student has to do and he or she does it. It in no way determines if the potential doctor actually is truly a compassionate soul. It also does not take into account that a student might be working at two jobs in order to pay for his premedical education and does not have the spare time to try to impress an admissions committee with contrived behavior. It would also do well to eliminate psychiatrists from the admissions committees. If anyone knows less about the type of person that is needed to practice good, compassionate medicine on a day by day basis, it is a psychiatrist. None of them actually know what is required of a doctor beset by numerous needs of patients and how to organize his or her day in order to accomplish the smooth process of never appearing frustrated. This failure of medical schools to recognize this behavioral trend that now fully encompasses medicine, and to do something about it, is creating a void that medicine is oozing in, slowly and relentlessly. This attitude is far more dangerous to medicine than the earlier attitudes of showing how much money they were accruing.

Chapter 14

Life After Retirement — True Great Discoveries Come Out of the Blue

After my wife Betty was able to get Mercy Medical accredited, she was a totally exhausted soul. The task had completely drained her physically and emotionally, and she would come home shedding tears over something that happened at work. This was about ten years before my retirement, and I began to think of something that she could do that would be something she liked but would have absolutely nothing to do with the nursing profession. Suddenly it dawned on me: we could open an antique shop, which would keep her in one of her favorite pastimes. We knew as much about running an antique shop as Pap did about farming when he bought his farm. Again, the arrogance of ignorance was in full sway.

We decided to see about putting it in Fairhope, Alabama, because it was just beginning to be a trendy place. We found an old two-storied building on Fairhope Avenue, rented the bottom floor, and we were in business. Little did we know that the roof and walls leaked like a sieve. After a few heavy showers, we became expert at putting out big trash cans in the right spot to catch all the water coming through the ceiling. We even went to the trouble of getting an estimate for the cost for a new roof and repairing the leaky brick walls. When the contractor presented the proposed cost to the owner, he paled to the point that I was afraid he was going to have apoplexy. Of course the repairs didn't happen, and we persevered with trash cans until we moved at a later date. We would get beat-up old furniture, and I would restore it. That allowed us to sell it a little cheaper than our competition. We started taking in antiques for restoration and also sold some of my antique restorations. We started bringing in a little money, and then we were able to improve our merchandise. Betty was actually beginning to enjoy herself.

Somewhere in the time frame of still being in practice, I began to miss my music. I was a long way from being a competent pianist, and I didn't even have a trombone any more. So since Paul, John, and later, Valerie and Rhonda, all sang in the choir at church, I thought I might give it a try. I never became exceptional by any stretch of the imagination, but I could carry my bass part. I enjoyed this for many years before realizing that I was beginning to sing more than a little flat, and I went into self-imposed retirement. We had some great experiences because of our music.

About three years after Betty and I were married, the choir directors set up a choir tour in Europe for the Dauphin Way Methodist Church choir. For this, Betty decided to become a pseudo-Methodist. We went to Holland and then on into West Germany. The next day we went into East Germany, and found it to be just like the movies depicted it, except more so. When we returned to West Germany and Heidelberg, we got a message that Pap had died. We caught a plane back home and I very sadly buried my father.

One day Betty turned to me and exclaimed, "We need to move the kitchen sink." I told her that the sink was not a piece of furniture and it could not just be moved. It had things attached to it that needed to be removed. This ushered in the great remodeling of the back of the house. We got my old friend Tommy McCowan to come over and give us some ideas about adding on. We moved walls, took out doors, widened porches, and added a deck. To do this, Tommy hired a fellow to do the carpentry work and sub-contractors were employed to do electrical, plumbing, etc. The carpenter brought his nephew to help him and, after spending several thousands of dollars, we got the sink moved about four feet.

By the time the house re-modeler and his nephew had finished reworking the back of the house, they became very interested in learning my business of antique furniture restoration along with the building of antique reproductions. We moved the tools in Pap's shop to Mobile, and with the addition of his nephew, we started to make that part of the business grow. Betty decided to close the antique shop in Fairhope; the ride back and forth every day had begun to grind on her nerves.

The antique restoration and reproduction business began to grow exponentially. We were getting work from as far east as Charleston and Savannah, and as far west as San Diego. We made regular trips to Montgomery and sometimes Birmingham. The uncle eventually left to form his own business, but the nephew stayed, and work continued at the same pace. After I retired from the practice of medicine, I spent a lot more time there. Things went well for a long time, with a work force of six or seven men and women.

However, though the work continued, the income began to fall. It eventually came to light that the nephew had been stealing from me in astronomical amounts. In addition, he had been stealing furniture and several thousands of dollars' worth of rare Blue Willow china that Betty kept stored there. He was arrested, pleaded guilty, and now I'm getting paid about thirty-three dollars per month through the civil court in restitution. I fear it is going to take him many, many years at that rate. During this debacle I could not pay my taxes or bills because of the marked decrease in money flow. Valerie, using her CPA skills, got it all settled, though I had to close the business. All the time and effort talking with her about the need for an advanced education paid off. God bless her.

I was now down to just piddling in the shop, working puzzles in order to keep my mind from deterioration, and thinking. Of course we had our social obligations to meet. About two years ago, Betty and I went out of town to a wedding of one of our friend's sons. There was a brunch the morning of the wedding at a beautiful home of a friend of the bride. There I was introduced to a brother of the groom's mother who I wasn't aware existed. I knew that the groom's mother had a sister who was a lesbian, and she had another brother who was also gay. I didn't think too much about it after that.

Now Betty is a huge wedding fan, and when she is not directing them, she likes to go early so she can see everybody else come in. This is not my favorite sport, and while we were sitting there in the groom's section, the groom's lesbian aunt came in and sat directly in front of us, separated by two rows. Since I didn't have anything else to do, I just let my mind wander. I began to think of the groom's maternal ancestry and the fact that there were two boys and two girls, one of each sex being gay. I distinctly remember thinking,

"Isn't that something? Two girls and two boys and one of each are gay. Wait a minute; that is a Mendelian inheritance pattern." I turned to Betty and said with great excitement, "Betty, I've got it figured out. Homosexuality is an inherited condition."

Despite my obvious excitement, all she would say was, "I can't talk to you now; we are at a wedding."

When I got back to Mobile, I called Wladimir and discussed my thoughts. He became as excited about it as I, and we began looking into it. After seven years of collecting data from a lot of questionnaires and collecting individual family trees for the presence of homosexuality, we have come to the inescapable fact that homosexuality is definitely an inherited condition. It is inherited as a recessive gene that requires both parents to be a carrier of a homosexual trait. Excessive genes are not a rare thing in medicine; cystic fibrosis, sickle cell anemia, blue eyes, and many other familial entities are inherited in the same manner When these parents who both have a recessive homosexual trait have children, mathematically the offspring would be one child having a match of recessive homosexual traits, two being carriers with one normal trait and one recessive homosexual trait, and one child having two heterosexual traits. If they begot sufficient numbers of children it would eventually work out that way, but it just doesn't happen that precisely in real life. Recessive trait parents may have only one affected child within families with no known identified homosexuals for generations. In our data, about forty percent of homosexual informers fell into this category. The remainder of our informants had many homosexual male and female siblings and homosexual ancestors both close and distant. Homosexuals had very few homosexual children. A very interesting piece of our data arose from our detailed family histories. When lesbians bore children, no matter where he fell in the birth order of offspring, the first born male was always a homosexual. I have no hypothesis that explains this. Our findings showing homosexuality is a familial entity has been submitted for publication.

Other investigators are looking into the selection of same-sex mates on a molecular level. The brain functions solely by chemicals. Neurotransmitters cause behavioral patterns, and they are being scrutinized as to their role in inherited basic behavior. One of these most basic behavioral patterns in mammals is the selection of a sexual preference when reproductive hormones begin to appear at puberty. The neurotransmitter, 5-hydroxytriptamine (5HT) has been shown to have control of sexual behavior of male mice and humans. Studies, so far only reported in mice, have revealed that a male mouse, genetically bred to manufacture low levels of 5HT, when placed in a cage with male and female mice will mount the male mouse. Thirty-five minutes after receiving an injection on 5HT to raise the blood level to normal, the mouse leaves the male mate and begins to mount the female. This allows us to form an operating hypothesis that what a homosexual inherits is an inability to make 5HT because of missing or defective enzymes or an abnormal 5HT. This results in low levels of 5HT in the homosexual offspring. There is a great deal of exciting work to be done here. I am afraid that the young folks are going to have the fun of proving or disproving this hypothesis.

There have now been two very exciting things that have come my way since my retirement. They have kept my thinking active and alert. I am truly glad that I didn't just ignore the opportunities presented to me with my sudden recognition of homosexuality of being inherited, nor the pleasant discovery of "Victoria's mixture." It is a good feeling to still be worth something.

As I sit here writing these final words of this book, I realize that I am only assuming that these latter projects are over for me when I get them all published. That is the beauty of life; it is so exciting to try to determine what the next program really is. I know that I have had an impelling feeling to finish this book. I have never had a desire to write until now, and I feel no desire to write anything else other than my scientific articles. All of us will have to wait and see.

Chapter 15

Musings of an Old Coot, Codger, or Fool — It All Depends on Perspective

This chapter was originally meant to be some mixture of advice, observations, and things that I had become aware of in my rather long life and wanted to pass along to my grandchildren and great-grandchildren. It occurred to me that you, the reader, might enjoy reading through these thoughts, too. I don't have an awful lot of advice to give. I would recommend one of my favorite pieces of advice given to me, *Keep small things small.*

When I look at the present generation, I see a lot of people with no patience. It is the time in which we live; everything has to be done in a hurry. Fast food, fast cars, must get to my destination in a hurry (for what?), and can't stay put in one place doing one thing at a time are all symptoms of this "hurry" syndrome. The main problem with this is that there is no time to appreciate what you have in this world. The only thing that really matters is having food to eat, comfortable shelter, and the love of your family. That sometimes is the hardest to acquire. Never become worshipers of things; they can be lost in an instant.

If you undertake something that is important and worthwhile in your eyes, it will be the most fulfilling thing you will ever undertake. If you keep your eyes and ears open, the opportunities will make themselves obvious if you will just respond to them.

When you do accept these opportunities, the obvious thing that caused you to take that particular course may not be evident at first, or even immediately afterward, but eventually the picture will become clear as to why you undertook the original task. For instance, I have thought many times as to why I became entangled with South Alabama. I didn't answer any particular need, nor did I accomplish something great by being there. One day, while pondering my findings with Wladimir, it hit me. If I hadn't done that job, I wouldn't have Wladimir for this riddle of homosexuality. See what I mean? There's no reason to get in a hurry, things that have meaning sometimes move at a snail's pace.

If any of you elect medicine as a profession, you will not experience many or most of the things that I have in my lifetime. I believe that all of the professions have, to some extent, lost their reason for being, some more so than others. If you define a profession as what people pursue as a vocation that is done for the public good, then there are not many professions left. Medicine, law, teaching, and journalism have all essentially become trades and now have a business approach instead of a humanistic approach. All have put their own desires and their comfort far ahead of the public good.

I have given a lot of thought to this demise of medicine as a profession. It is not that there are no physicians of the old school left, but they are becoming more and more rare. As I have mentioned earlier, there appears to be a trend now for physicians to work an eight-hour day. That type of day does not have time for time-consuming things such as giving IV fluids, suturing wounds, or giving IV medications. Doing these things would involve not being able to leave the office at 5:00 p.m. All such patients are admitted to the emergency room, where they are taken care of by busy, rushed physicians with very little training in pediatrics.

There the patients sit for long periods of time, waiting for someone to take care of them or their child, when they just left the office of the physician who had already agreed to take care of them or their child. If a physician accepts someone as a patient, then he or she, or the immediate partner, should take care of the patient to the bitter end or else refer them to a specialist who has some special skill to solve the problem. In pediatrics, this referral should be done only after speaking to the specialist and telling him or her what the diagnosis is and what procedure needs to be done.

The practice of sending people from the doctor's office to the emergency room drastically increases the cost of medical care. There, the patient is being cared for by someone who has to start all over to determine what the problem is and then start the initial therapy. All of this is carried on in an atmosphere of a business enterprise in which there are enormous charges for everything, including the little box of tissues that might be used. To this, add the fact that the vast majority of emergency physicians have the personality of working hard and enjoying it, but want to have nothing to do with any type of follow-up care, Thus the patient has to trudge back to the "doctor" who was too busy to take care of the patient in the beginning. Now, add to that plight the huge number of individuals who have no regular physician to care for them and go to the emergency rooms for their primary care. If all of these patients could have a physician who really meant it when he or she accepted them as a new patient and would provide care after 5:00 p.m., think of the improvement in patient care and health care costs. One of the first things needed is to remove all but the true emergencies out of the hospitals. Then care could be given at a much lower costs because the institution doesn't have to assume some of the costs of such things as open heart surgery that insurance doesn't adequately cover. All kinds of ways come to mind as to how medical care could be given at times other than regular office hours, and not by giving the patient an office appointment to come in in three weeks. It starts with, "The patient always comes first."

There are several things that have severely changed the way that medicine is practiced on a day-to-day basis. As I have tried to explain to you in this book, many things have happened through the years to change medicine. The first is the explosion of subspecialties in the various branches of medicine. Always remember Parkinson's first law. I readily admit that I was one of the people who saw a need for this, and we set up educational teaching programs to accomplish this. However, this pendulum has swung too far in this direction. Now we have a plethora of clinicians who have developed very limited skills and knowledge except in a narrow slice of medicine. This has resulted in the poor patient continually being shuffled between physicians, each with limited knowledge. The physician with good general knowledge is needed to put all the limited knowledge together and end the travels and waiting room stays for the sick patient. This individual is not showing up at the present time. Rather, presently if a patient presents himself for diagnosis and treatment, the pediatrician or internist starts the insanity of constant referrals. I personally believe that it is a problem of laziness in which the physician doesn't want to expend the energy and time to do most of the investigations himself or herself, and the always constant fear of litigation where he or she can be accused of practicing beyond his or her competence. A lot of common sense leadership is needed here.

There are really only two main divisions of medicine, the diagnostic or medical branch and the technical or surgical branch. I found through my academic years that I could accurately predict the field of medicine that each student would choose as a medical career based on personality and academic standing in their class. Their personalities dictate their choice between what Dr. Tinsley Harrison called "the thinkers" and "the doers." He always said the doers make surgeons. If you contemplate what it is that causes a physician to be considered a superb surgeon, it is not his extensive knowledge about the details of a clinical condition. It is his mastery of surgical techniques that makes that individual outstanding. Yet potential residents are never screened for manual dexterity, which is an inherited and not a taught thing. This leads to many surgical types who were described to me by Dr. John Kirkland, the renowned cardiovascular surgeon, as "operating as if they were using their feet." Many enter the surgical fields, few are outstanding. Their academic achievements then tend to separate these students into their chosen subspecialties. Of course, not all students fall into this overall picture, but the vast majority do. Essentially all of the surgical subspecialties come out of the lower third of the class, this includes ENT, orthopedics, urology, proctology, and, yes, neurosurgery. General surgeons usually arrive from the middle third, and cardiovascular and thoracic surgeons from the top third. This leaves us with a large group of highly trained technical people with very limited knowledge of anything in medicine outside their very narrow discipline. It is imperative that the "thinkers" refer their patients for a special technical chore and little else.

The obstetrics and gynecologists generally come from the middle third and the upper part of the lower third of thc class academically. The males are usually snappy dressers and are attractive to women. The females are ordinarily very plain dressers with little use of cosmetics to improve their appearance. Because of so much litigation associated with the birthing of babies, the majority of these specialists drop the obstetrical part of their practice leaving fewer and fewer physicians to bear this load.

The remaining thinkers divide themselves also by their academic achievements and their personalities. For some reason, unfathomable by me, ophthalmologists essentially all come from the top ten percent of every class. In my experience they are always pleasant, calm, likeable, and very efficient in their chosen field. Dermatologists also tend to come from the upper third or the top of the middle third. They are bright, efficient, and knowledgeable because many diseases first symptoms occur on the skin. They also don't have a desire to take care of a patient's total health care; they don't want to work hard; and they want to make money. The students in the upper and high-middle-third of their class standings who don't particularly like dealing with people generally go into pathology or radiology. The psychiatrists come from all levels and are generally shown to be individuals who have personality problems and are searching for an understanding of themselves. Neurologists tend to come from the middle third and tend to be stodgy people.

The remaining physicians from the upper and middle-thirds are made up of internists, pediatricians, and family practice doctors. As a general rule, they are competent, pleasant and generally very good physicians in the professional sense of the word. Internal medicine doctors tend to be very serious about their work, and they frequently have been known to make morning hospital rounds without ever smiling. They do have a tendency to feel a little superior to their pediatric and family practice comrades, which always has amused me. I've repeatedly said that I would rather surrender the care of a pediatric patient to a surgeon than an internist, because an internist only thinks in terms of degenerating tissue. In pediatrics, doctors think in terms of growing, vibrant tissue, not degenerating.

Thus the graduating physicians each year divide themselves into the various medical groups that have prevailed for generation after generation. The problem is that only a few of the pediatric and family groups are doing what they are best suited for, i.e., delivering medical care to the general public in municipalities and rural areas and referring to specialists only when they need technical help. Since these graduating students have zero exposure to a very competent medical practice in the primary care fields, they never discover the fact that taking care of patients is an enormous amount of fun. Taking care of ninety to ninety-five of all the problems that occur with your patients is extremely enjoyable. I know; I did it for years. I understand that it requires long hours, but doing it is not drudgery when you are truly enjoying it.

There are two things which must change before this is possible again. The first is that medical schools have to realize that their brightest and best need to be taught that being an excellent clinician is something that should be strived for. To accomplish this, the good clinicians should again assume their rightful place of being the most admired of the clinical faculty members, and not the myopic superspecialist. The second thing is that physicians on the forefront of medical care should have tort reform that allows them to take care of the most of their patients' problems without an unneeded referral to a subspecialist with limited knowledge in order to stymie a potential lawsuit.

If any of you do enter the practice of medicine, remember that no greater honor can be given to a physician than a person voluntarily giving themselves, or a member of their family, to your medical care. They, in essence, are telling you that you have all their trust, respect, and confidence in your willingness to get the job done to the best of your ability. If a fellow doctor turns himself or his or her family member, especially his or her children, to your care, that is the highest compliment that you will ever receive.

The most dangerous things that you can become involved with are egotism, greed, and selfishness. If you have children, make sure that you put their good above anything that you as their parent might yearn for yourself. Remember, they did not ask to be born, and you, as their parent, must ensure their education to whatever level it takes to ensure their chosen life's work. Also, remember no two children are the same, regardless of the fact that they share a lot of the same genes as their siblings. To educate and guide your children requires a lot of parental sacrifice. Be prepared to give it freely; if you can't, then you shouldn't have children.

Sooner or later, you have to decide what to do with your life. Don't make the mistake of deciding to be poor. Many people make this choice without realizing it by knowingly making the decision to not learn a skill. You get paid by the level of various skills that you have. If your skill is the same as thousands of others, then there is not going to be anyone beating down the door to hire you. The level of pay follows these same guidelines. If you can't do more than thousands of people, then the level of pay will be low. Your earning ability rises at the same rate as the scarcity of your accumulated skills and knowledge. In other words, the fewer people one has to compete against to fill a job requirement, the higher will be the salary offered. This leads us to one more of my father's jokes. This retired maintenance man was sleeping very soundly one night when his phone rang. It was the factory where he had worked for many years. It seems that one of the huge machines wouldn't run and no one could get it started. They pleaded with him to come look at it, so he slowly crawled out of bed and made his way over to the plant. After looking at the machine for a few minutes, he reached down, picked up a hammer, and gave a projection a sharp rap. The machine roared into action, and the old man picked up his tools and went home. Later the factory received a bill from him for ten thousand dollars. They wrote back and said that the price seemed excessive and would like an itemized bill. In the return mail came a bill which said: "Hitting with hammer: $1.50. Knowing where to hit: $9,998.50."

Go out and decide what you want to do with your life. Take all the time that you need, for this is one of the most important decisions you will make. There is nothing worse than working all of your life at a profession or trade that you despise. It will lead to a miserable existence. Once you decide on your occupational future, learn all you can about it and make yourself indispensable. Your life will be full, and what's more, you will be happy in your work.

Remember that money, and what it can buy, are not worth the effort it takes to achieve. Trying to keep up with the Joneses is a perfect example of the three dangers listed above. In my practice of pediatrics, I saw more patients per day with the most time-consuming diseases of anyone in the group yet I put less money on the books than anyone. We always had a daily steady stream of patients coming in the back door. I mentioned it to Betty, and she said that I wouldn't have been me if I had done it differently.

In my workshop, ever so often one of my old leukemia patients drops in to see me. When she was a child, we had a tough trip getting her leukemia under control and she required a lot of extra therapy. She went on to become a nurse, got married, and then had the heartbreak of her husband being unfaithful and abandoning her. Still, she always appears upbeat. She still comes around, hugs my neck like she did as a child, and tells me that she loves me. The last time I saw her, she told me, "I always come to see you on my birthday." Trust me, money cannot buy that feeling.

Epilogue

About thirty years ago, Dr. Haydn Childs, the medical director of Providence Hospital in Mobile, Alabama, called me and invited me to have lunch with him. He wanted to pick my brain as to what I thought was the future of the practice of medicine in the United States. I didn't have to think long about my answer because I was bemoaning that future in my own mind most of my waking hours. I told him that the United States was moving rapidly to the British system of medicine, where a physician would be on the medical staff and would be employed by the hospital to practice medicine the way that the hospital administration wanted it practiced. He later wrote me a letter saying that he totally disagreed with me and that medicine would never be under the control of hospital administrations.

I ran into Haydn at an alumni meeting when my class was celebrating the fifty-fifth anniversary of our graduation. I told him, "Haydn, do you remember our discussion of the future of medicine about thirty years ago?" He just smiled a sad smile and nodded his head.

Even earlier than this, I was having a discussion with Dr. Joe Volker along these same lines. He said something I have never forgotten, "The trouble with medicine is that they have turned the operation of their hospitals over to the business people, and the humanity is leaving it. The dentists have never done this, and thus they have maintained their practice of dentistry under their own control." This has proven to be so true.

Today, the "medical community" met with President Obama to discuss lowering medical costs. There were pharmaceutical